HIGH VIBE HABITS

BECAUSE HAPPINESS ISN'T A WAITING GAME, IT'S A CREATING GAME

NITHYA KARIA

Printed in the United States of America
Hardcover ISBN: 978-1-967703-01-2
Paperback ISBN: 978-1-967703-02-9
Library of Congress Control Number: 2025937780

Muse Literary Publishing
Send feedback to hello@museliterary.com
Special discounts for bulk sales are available, please contact operations@museliterary.com

To my children for being brilliant examples of how to live and love. And for reminding me that the greatest teachers are eternal students.

To G, you make my every day.

66

Everything is created twice, first in the mind and then in reality.

—Robin Sharma

Table of Contents

INTRODUCTION

"Can't I just enjoy my ice cream?"

My ten-year-old son looks at me with tears in his eyes, pleading for permission to relish the ice cream sandwich in his hand. He's been waiting all week to try this chocolate-on-chocolate dessert that he's certain exists nowhere else in the world.

I feel the sting of tears in my own eyes. His face, with its ice cream-stained lips, normally turned upward with glee, is turning downward. I'm instantly sorry because his words make me painfully aware of what I've just done. I've sucked the joy out of this experience. I had the best of intentions. As a mother, it's my habit to remind him to eat well and take care of himself. After a week of a typical vacation diet of French fries and dessert, my reflexes kicked in and I didn't stop to check them.

But my son was right. Once we make a decision, we should let ourselves enjoy it. I know I was coming from a place of love. I was teaching my son about health, but I was also teaching him how to deprive himself of joy. And that's a learned habit I did not want to pass down.

Have you ever denied yourself the chance to enjoy something? Downtime, an accomplishment, a gift, a sunset, a compliment, maybe even an ice cream? Rushing off, not being present, declining the chance to say yes to feeling good?

Habits are the things we do so regularly they become our autopilot. This is great when our habits serve us and not so great when they become obstacles to our goals. I'm here to explore how your current habits might be barriers to joy and how you can choose new habits and get proactive about your happiness instead, allowing yourself to eliminate stress and unlock the potential happiness around you with just five simple habits: the High Vibe Habits.

Consistency creates results. Have you ever felt the heart-warming sensation of writing a gratitude list only to find yourself a day or two later right back where you started? We reap the benefits of practices like this when we do them regularly. Why? Because they transform from a thing we do into a way we engage with the world. We rewire our brains and choose where we focus. And that means gratitude, and all wellness practices, are a lens through which we see our life. Not something we do, but a way we move through the world. This isn't about good or bad or wrong or right. It's the awareness that our habits have the power to help us find happiness as a reflex.

For many of us, the things we bring into our lives that are meant to bring us joy—like the items on our gratefulness list—end up depleting us instead. But even so, we're not looking to get rid of them, are we? We're looking for a way to find joy with them. To not lose ourselves in the life we create.

I want to be really clear. The habits I'm sharing with you aren't here to fix you. There's nothing wrong with you. We are all products of our environment, where our family, culture, and society have brought us up to practice what I call "learned deprivation." They've taken some of the natural tendencies that were designed to help us survive, like negativity and fear, and nurtured them to the point that they've become destructive habits. We have been encouraged to see the world and ourselves through a negative lens that we believe will motivate us to be better and have more.

But being more isn't created from feeling less. We are taught and praised for our capacity to give. But it's your capacity to receive that will unlock your best life yet. The High Vibe Habits are how you allow yourself to receive consistently.

I've been intimately familiar with less: not being enough, having enough, or doing enough. I pushed myself hard, linked stress and responsibility, and was rewarded for it. I had achieved just about everything I'd gone after—a good education, great jobs, a loving partner, and two healthy children. Asking to feel good on top of all of that felt ungrateful. But at my lowest, I'd also earned insomnia and fatigue and felt irritable, sad, and dull. Don't get me wrong, I was happy too, but that emotion didn't have the same stickiness as the other things.

I set the bar impossibly high. I was willing to do whatever it took to uphold the picture of perfection in my mind. And then judged myself worthy by whether I met my targets. I wanted to be the best everything I could be.

When I fell short, the answer was always to work harder, try harder, do more. But in the end, it didn't feel right. I was "with" my children but tearing up when Google Photos would send me a "remember this day" picture because I felt like I was missing out. I was physically present but mentally overloaded. My mind, body, happiness, and family were paying the price for perfection.

I began to wonder if maybe I just wanted too much. But being driven is a part of my DNA. I didn't want to stop dreaming; I wanted to figure out how to live a life I felt good about and that made me feel good. I knew that stress and joy couldn't coexist within me, but could achievement and joy? Did I have to wait to be happy and feel good after the work was done, the goals were met, and the life was lived?

The answer? Joy isn't a destination; it's in every step of the journey. . .

I didn't always feel as comfortable as I do now with being *un*comfortable. It's not that I don't care what other people think, say, or feel about me, it's that I care more about what *I* think and feel about the life I'm living.

When feeling good became a primary goal, I began to see just how much time I was spending feeling poorly. Comparison, judgment, guilt, obligation, regret—all the things that I believed were pushing me forward were holding me back. When feeling good became one of my success metrics, it let me re-evaluate almost everything in my life. Words like *failure, perfect, enough, worthy, should,* and *need* have new meanings, some disappearing from my vocabulary completely.

Life is neutral—we create meaning. Do you believe that? We are responsible for our life experiences. That can feel scary or empowering; it's your choice. While it's not easy to question the "truths" we live by, it's essential if we want a constructive perspective. A rainy wedding day is considered by some to be good luck, a blessing. But for someone else, it would be disastrous. For others still, an inconvenience. Who's right? All of them. What we believe in our minds becomes our reality.

Why High Vibe Habits?

Look around your life. I have no doubt that your current habits have brought a lot of great things into your life. Well done! But like me, you may have also picked up a few less desirable habits like comparison, judgment, and guilt that never let you be, have, or do enough. I'm proud of what I've accomplished, but what I noticed was that so-called "good" habits can also create "bad" outcomes. Working hard is great, but not if you never allow yourself to rest. All the great habits I cultivated in my youth focused on my capacity to give, but none of them taught me how to receive. Achievement is about how much you give. Happiness is about how much you allow yourself to receive.

Joy (and all the other high-vibrational emotions) is expansive. It's a state that can't be contained. Feeling good compels you to share the overflow of energy. Think about it. When you feel good, what do you do? How much do you get done? How much easier does life feel? How much more enjoyable is it? I bet you smile, give compliments, offer to do things for people and go the extra mile with ease. I found five simple habits that offered me everything I needed because they

7

pointed me to the one thing I wanted: happiness.

Success, the kind that gets you good grades, into great schools, and lands you dream jobs, seemed to have a simple enough formula. It was all based on my ability to pour into passions, projects, and people. Hard work, perseverance, tenacity, attitude. I could see a formula for success, and I was achieving it.

But what about a formula for happiness? In my heart, I believed in the strength of it. But in reality, there was a fragility to it. Happiness had to be earned and was swallowed whole by my anxiety and stress. I walked on eggshells and lived a life where I checked all the boxes by pleasing and creating a life that others applauded and appreciated. Truth be told, I didn't want to get rid of what I'd brought into my life (spouse, kids, career, friendships). *I wanted to enjoy it all.* I wanted to feel enough. I wanted to stop making decisions to prove my worth. I wanted to feel smart, capable, beautiful, and all the other things I'd at least partially denied myself. And the High Vibe Habits have offered me all that and more.

I tried just changing what I did, but until I changed what I believed, I wasn't free of all the baggage. This drag is what's exhausting you, not your desires. I've stepped away from so many "shoulds" and stepped towards a life of my design. I've homeschooled my children, traveled the world, written this book, spoken on stages, and coached other women to find their way.

I went through the discomfort of diving inwards and reprogramming my own beliefs so I could be my ally. The journey I'm sharing with you is how I went from believing I needed to squeeze more *in,* to my new goal of practicing how to squeeze more *out* of life. I distilled that process down and found the formula I'd been looking for—a way to make joy my reflex. And that's how the High Vibe Habits were born.

I assumed that all this happiness was going to cost me my productivity. But something surprising happened. This mental reorganization helped me shed my feelings of lack and fear of failure and opened me up to dreaming bigger and achieving more than I'd ever imagined possible. Feeling good is a worthy goal all by itself. But I can guarantee it will also bring you so much more.

As adults, we've come to accept a certain order about life. Dessert comes after dinner. Leisure comes after work. Just like that, joy, fun, and all the good stuff for me came after all the work was done. But what happens when the work is never done? When the to-do list is never-ending? We run off the assumption (because we're taught to) that time is meant for toiling, working, producing, sacrificing, and losing. But at what cost?

Nearly one-fifth of the American population suffers from mental health issues. And the onset of those is getting younger and younger[1]. Depression, anxiety, and chronic diseases (like heart attack, stroke, and diabetes) are consuming people's lives in increasing numbers[2]. Stress is a major contributor to each of those destructive diseases. We're unhappy with the way we

---

[1] Adult Prevalence of Mental Illness (AMI) 2022. Mental Health America. "Adult Data 2022," n.d. chrome-extension://efaidnbmnnnibpcajpcglclefindmkaj/https://mhanational.org/wp-content/uploads/2025/03/2022-State-of-Mental-Health-in-America.pdf

[2] Stuckler, David. "Population Causes and Consequences of Leading Chronic Diseases: A Comparative Analysis of Prevailing Explanations." *The Milbank Quarterly* 86, no. 2 (June 1, 2008): 273–326. https://onlinelibrary.wiley.com/doi/abs/10.1111/j.1468-0009.2008.00522.x

feel, the way we look, and the way our lives look. As a population, we're unhappy. Period.

The things we're used to bragging about and being praised for (working eighty-hour work weeks, barely sleeping, sacrificing our needs) are killing us, but equally as disturbing, they're robbing us of the joyful experience of living. Even when we do stop to question the sanity of this, we see everyone else living the same way. Our hearts grow heavy and our light dims without a clear way out. I speak from experience here. You can pour into your life, but if you don't let it pour back into you, you can have it all and still feel empty.

No one has the life they love by accident. Whether they realize it or not, they prioritize what matters. Happy and healthy people aren't that way by accident. It's not easier or more convenient for them. They prioritize what it takes to be happy and healthy. And those thoughts and actions become their *habits.*

Why High Vibe? You can't be in two places at once. And by being in this elevated state, it automatically means you're out of the lower-vibe emotions of fear, anxiety, worry, guilt, regret, shame, and judgment. It gets rid of stress, improves our health and energy, increases our confidence and productivity, lets us connect more deeply with others, and gives us more time. It changes the way we see ourselves, our lives, and everyone in it through a lens of love. This one goal improves our overall quality of life. It's the answer to everything I want: to be my best self and live my best life.

So how do we learn to carve out space in our full lives for how we really want to be living? Make time for what we actually want to be doing? You're about to find out.

In this book, I'll explore each of the High Vibe Habits with you: clarity, control, confidence, curiosity, and creativity. Clarity is where you begin to make your life your own. It will help you know where you're headed and how to get there. Control allows you to always stay in the driver's seat. Confidence lets you feel good about your choices and helps you keep making aligned ones. Curiosity and creativity are healthy habits to reflect on what comes your way and how to navigate it.

Maybe you want to find more joy in the life you have. Maybe you want to completely change things up. It doesn't matter because a habit is a way of showing up. It's a default mechanism. And when that mechanism is supportive of your needs and desires, you'll make decisions that always bring you closer to the life you want. I'm not promising you a perfect life. But I can guarantee you this: a compass and a map to always find your way back to feeling good.

This book is designed to be a multiplier in your life. It will help you thrive. It's going to amplify what you already have and open you up to create more. It's also an insurance plan. You've been working hard to create a lifestyle, a family, and a career that you want. This ensures you not only get to keep it but enjoy it. You get to stop doing more and start doing something different.

I went on a journey that began over a decade ago, looking to live the life I wanted. I devoured personal development and brain science books, got certified as a health coach, studied positive psychology and positive intelligence, and grounded all of that with spiritual growth work. I invested in myself and my future big-time, hiring coaches, joining masterminds, and attending wellness conferences. I shifted from trying to do all the things and feeling like I was losing myself and my sanity, to realizing it did not *all* matter to me. I quit thinking I was less for not doing more. When I looked at others, I let their lives be proof of possibility rather than my lack. A move from imitation to inspiration.

'Happily Ever After' starts with happily right now. I started with the smallest steps, basically wondering how I could make my day feel like a win. And then the next day, and the next. I realized questions like, "How could I not feel guilty for a coffee date instead of getting work done?" "How could I find time to do fifteen minutes of yoga before I picked the kids up from school?" "How could I enjoy my hair appointment instead of squeezing it in between errands and feeling rushed?" were clues to everyday ways I deprived myself of feeling good. Small choice after small choice I was reclaiming my power to create the experience I wanted.

Habits are the decision-makers that change the course of our lives. New decisions require new information (feelings and beliefs). Instead of trying to make more time, we'll look at how you allocate your resources (like time, money, and energy) in the first place. You might be surprised to find out it doesn't all need doing. I had to learn and accept several new concepts, beginning with the simplest: *It matters what you believe.* Thoughts determine your emotions. Emotions guide your choices. Choices create your life.

The Current Landscape

Let's do a mini realignment. Time isn't the enemy. Ask anyone who's been on the planet for a while, and they'll tell you that *time is a gift.* Time to laugh with friends, love on grandchildren, watch a sunset, and hold a hand: Each and every experience we get is a bonus. There are plenty of people who do not get these opportunities.

Why do we find ourselves busy and not doing the things that we want to do? The truth? Our calendars get eaten up by the expectation of who we're supposed to be. If you're busy living the life someone else decides for you, you're missing out on the one you want. High Vibe Habits don't just offer you the way to feeling good, they empower you to give yourself what you need.

Are you living at least one part of your life in a waiting sequence? Are you waiting for the right partner to make you feel loved? Waiting for more experience to feel confident instead of an imposter? Waiting for the right job to make you feel worthy? Most of us carry around the belief that the answer lies *outside* of us. The truth is the opposite. When you wait for a good grade to make you feel smart or the salary to say you're successful, you're missing the opportunity to gift yourself. What if you knew how to offer yourself the very thing you've been waiting for? If we're deciding who we are and what's possible for us based on what someone else thinks, we're also at their mercy if they change their minds. It matters what you believe. What we offer ourselves, we get to keep forever. The answer is *in*side.

A note of caution: If your brain is telling you there will be a better time, a right time, to prioritize feeling good: Something's always giving.

Yep, even when you feel like you're doing it all, especially when you think you're doing it all, something is giving. If it's not the laundry or the house, it might be your health or your joy. Each of us chooses where to spend our energy. I believe we want our lives to feel like more than a juggling act. That kind of life isn't sustainable. Or joyful. Or healthy. When your life doesn't make space for your needs, you're likely to end up burnt out, resentful, or both. High Vibe Habits are the way to keep giving (because they let you give back to yourself as well).

Your habits got you to where you are today. My five habits will help you prioritize your well-being with consistency and without guilt. What happens when you feel in control? You get to decide what you accept in your life. You get to decide what stays, what goes, what you want, and what you no longer accept. What's enough and what's still to come. You stop waiting for someone or something else to be the answer. The life that lights you up is waiting for you to claim it. The goal to thrive is a unique journey that will ask you to make a stand for yourself. It will require that you do things that not everyone else will value, support, or agree with. Equip yourself with the habits that make the journey possible and enjoyable.

Every word on these pages is meant to offer you hope, support, information, compassion, courage, or whatever else you need for where you are. You will not find any judgment, comparison, or guilt-inducing ideas. Without doing more, the High Vibe Habits bring down the barriers to joy that you've unknowingly built.

I know there are days when it feels like your life has swallowed you up and happiness is nowhere to be found. But I promise it hasn't vanished. Happiness didn't disappear from your life; it's just become less available. Why?

Habits.

You've been practicing a set of habits that have you focused on the gap. And you can practice a set of habits to readjust your focus. Wherever you are, you're only a few habits away from a life that feels different. If you don't let yourself receive, you hold yourself back from giving and living your absolute best.

Many things require time and patience, but happiness isn't one of them. Are you ready to get rid of those barriers you've built? Joy is waiting for you and so am I. Let's do this.

"

You have always had the power, dear;
you just had to learn it for yourself.

—*Glinda the Good Witch*

ONE

UNLEARNING

Threadbare.

That's the word I used to describe myself at that point. I was doing it all but barely holding it together inside. There was physical fatigue (as if I'd just hiked ten miles), and there was mental fatigue; two very different animals. Both left me exhausted, but the mental clutter was overwhelming. It was the kind of tiredness that was never resolved with a better night's sleep or even less work. Its only remedy was clarity.

That Monday morning, I awoke buzzing with anticipation. Today marked a big day. We were finally getting a backsplash put in our kitchen. It's not that backsplashes are that big of a deal, but we had finally decided to invest in our home so we could enjoy it right now, regardless of whether we sold it or not. It was business as usual, with my husband, Gautam, biking to work and me shuttling school drop-off. The tile guy showed up and had just got to work when my husband's number popped up on my phone. Assuming he was checking in with the tile job, I excitedly answered.

"I'm okay. . . but I was just hit by a car. I'm going to walk to the office and get checked out."

The shock put me in an out-of-body experience. "Go to the emergency room," I heard myself firmly saying. Gautam sounded totally fine except for the fact that he seemed more concerned about locking up his bike than getting himself to the hospital. I urged him again and he went—after he locked up his bike at the office.

I left my house to the very kind gentleman tiling our kitchen and ran to the car. I don't remember the drive downtown, but I kept holding on to the sound of Gautam's voice. It was reassurance that he was okay even though he'd been hit by a car. I slid into a parking spot by the Northwestern ER downtown and braced myself. I didn't linger on any one of the millions of thoughts racing through my mind. I was too busy making sure that the dam blocking my emotions held up. The automatic doors slid open, and a gust of cold air immediately gave me the chills.

The phones were ringing and there was a strong smell of urine as I walked up to the front desk. The volunteer confirmed that Gautam was inside but alerted me that I'd have to wait until he got the okay from inside before I could enter. There were ill people, injured people, and homeless people in almost every chair. I stood by the door for a few minutes before I got the all-clear.

As soon as the doors were unlocked, my eyes were scanning the area. The yellow of the lights cast a jaundiced glow on everything. A police officer stood in front of one room, his radio going off in spurts. I kept walking since there was no one to assist me, glancing from room to room. I got to the back of the U-shaped hallway and saw him.

There he was, waiting for an x-ray on an examination table with his leg, or at least what was supposed to be his leg, stretched out. It was in one piece, but with his pants cut open, its bizarre shape, and the blood, it looked like a Halloween prop. He smiled at me and the floodgates opened.

I stepped outside while he completed his X-rays and wept. They were tears of joy, fear, sadness, anger, relief, and uncertainty. Later, he would tell me that someone had made an illegal right turn, knocking him off his bike and into oncoming traffic, where a delivery truck then ran over his leg. He would eventually describe this event as "unlucky." But also, how lucky had we been? Had the whole scene been shifted a few feet, our lives would've been changed forever.

Over the next few weeks, I told almost no one. I'd never recoiled from friendship in this way, but I didn't know where to begin. The weird thing was it seemed easier to spill my guts to total strangers than it did to tell my best friends. Each day felt the same. I woke from a heavy sleep to prep the kids for school and get my husband settled. The downstairs couch became his new domain.

Because I told myself "I'm not someone who sacrifices quality," I still fixed food from scratch, while brewing special healing herbal teas and doing three roundtrips to get the kids to and from school. I hung onto my neuroses like my life depended on them— like if I budged an inch on the details, everything would come crashing down.

The initial accident was hard, but its aftermath was life-altering for me. His immobility left me a caretaker and single parent for weeks. I found a routine to manage it all, but I can still remember feeling so guilty for what was building up inside me. I hadn't taken the time to identify what exactly it was, only that I was beginning to feel like a pressure cooker. I was caring for his physical needs, but I was not able to provide emotional support or love. It was easier to hand him dinner than it was to hug him.

I desperately needed a break. I managed to meet a friend for a quick, early bite around the corner from my house. Empanada in hand, my friend asked me, "What would help? You keep saying there's too much to do, but what can you delegate?" I'd had people offer me a meal, a shoulder to cry on, but no one had offered to problem-solve with me yet. My voice cracked as we talked through things. It was bizarre how I wasn't able to identify what I needed help with. There was the house, the cooking, the schlepping, the parenting, but I couldn't give any of that up.

"I don't have the energy to research a cleaning service or figure out a carpool solution," I heard myself say.

As I talked through things, I realized those didn't seem to be the problem. They were just busyness, the physical fatigue. And then I heard myself talking about my fears, my ill-preparedness, my desire for more. Where was all of this coming from?

The idea of losing everything in an instant made my once-solid life feel so fragile. All of it could change in a second. This total loss of control left me feeling like a mere passenger in my own life. And now, the Ghost of Christmas Future was visiting me, showing me a glimpse of what my life might look like decades down the road. Performing a bunch of functions isn't living. A checked-off to-do list isn't living inspired. Checking obligatory boxes doesn't necessarily lead us to our purpose. The things we *do* are tiring. But the things we *think* either sink our souls or let us soar. Hitting the bottom can be good for something. It can move us from fear into curiosity. If there was no guarantee in life, what did I have to lose if I let go of what life was "supposed" to look like and went after what felt good? I began to question everything because I was seeing it all from a new perspective.

A lifetime of giving and living for others, taking just the scraps for myself, was going to leave me a ghost in my own life, slowly fading from vibrancy into a shadow of myself. In the end, no job, man, friend, destination, accolade, or event could give me what I wanted. Someone or something else was never the answer.

I was doing was doing the work for the things I wanted: family, a loving marriage, happy and healthy kids, opportunity, and financial freedom. I was grateful and appreciative of all of it. I was committed to all of it. But that perspective got drowned out daily. I was stuck seeing what wasn't in my life and what still needed doing and that left me feeling poorly. Where was there space for how I felt? Where did I fit into my life? For the longest time, I had believed that feeling low vibe was a sign I was on the right path, that I was doing enough. But I wanted to feel something radically different. I wanted to engage with my life in a way that let me tap into positive emotions. I knew how to achieve, I knew how to work hard, but I couldn't see an alternative path. I genuinely and almost desperately wanted to know, *what am I missing?* Turns out the answer was simple—I was missing countless opportunities to feel good because it was my habit to feel bad.

I was used to depriving myself of receiving from the life I was living because I grew up believing that feeling good was something to earn. Stop feeling bad on your way to feeling good. We all want to feel good. We might each call it by a different name: successful, peaceful, wealthy, healthy, purposeful. But everything we do; we do with the end desire to feel good. What you might not have realized though is that your current habits might actually be blocking you from achieving your end goal. Yep, that's right. You might be creating the barriers you're working so hard to maneuver around.

Have you ever suffered from something painful or really uncomfortable? Muscle spasms, nerve pain, migraines, or even something like an injured wrist? Think about how difficult it made it to go about your day. Did it make you more irritable, influence your decisions, and demand your attention? Has it ever made you want to shut out the world until you feel better? I've been there and all my thoughts channeled the same desire: Make it go away. And even though we have to go on with our lives, the pain demands our attention. Our focus is narrowed.

Pain—physical or emotional—is a distraction. Low vibrational states like sadness, worry, jealousy, or anger also narrow our focus. We tend to zone in on what we aren't, what we don't have, and what we'll never have. We use this lens on ourselves and other people. We do this because all those not-so-great feelings create stress. When we live in these low-vibe emotions day after day, we create chronic stress. Neuroendocrinology researcher and professor Robert Sapolsky explains how chronic stress negatively affects our anterior cingulate cortex (ACC), which diminishes what our brains are capable of in all sorts of vital areas of life. Areas like empathy, working memory, tolerance, generosity, and judgment are adversely affected, which means that we are making it harder to achieve the things we want most in life—things like success, deep connection, and happiness[3].

---

[3] *Dr. Robert Sapolsky – The Shocking New Science of How to Manage Your Stress,* Modern Wisdom podcast Episode 693, October 14, 2023.

No doubt, many of us have created a lot in our lives while not feeling good. You may not have been bothered by how you are motivated, as long as you're producing the right result. But as I just pointed out, if you are living in states of chronic stress, you can't be performing at your best. What you've accomplished so far is amazing. Now, think about what's still to come when you work from high-vibe states. Being motivated by fear is not the same as being inspired by possibility. Drive can be created by possibility instead of lack. It's easy to believe that our emotions aren't a problem if we are high-functioning humans. But that thing we're still chasing—balance, ease, fulfillment—only makes itself available from an alternate, high-vibe perspective.

To embrace new habits means letting go of old ones. The High Vibe Habits are already a part of you. The work will be to begin to rely on them, to trust them, and to override your reflex to turn to a less constructive one. This rewiring process is called *unlearning*.

If I told you that you couldn't be in LA and New York at the same time, you'd get it.

---

https://podcasts.apple.com/dk/podcast/693-dr-robert-sapolsky-the-shocking-new-science-of/id1347973549?i=1000631283709

But the same goes for our beliefs and emotions. Stress includes a variety of emotions that don't always seem obvious. Things like worry, sadness, frustration, and anything that shifts you out of feeling good can induce a stress response in your body. High Vibe Habits transform your old stress habits into more productive habits. You'll learn to gather the information emotions offer you. They let you focus on and align with your values and goals so you can actually reach them *and* feel good.

I can't tell you how many women I know who end up feeling bad on their way to feeling good. I've been there. I have beat myself up and felt disappointed in myself for not being able to maintain an impossible standard. Or even someone else's perfectly *normal* standard. But when how you feel about yourself and your life is relative to someone else, you give away the power to offer yourself what you need.

Unlearning is putting the power to control how you experience life back into your hands. In some general sense, we're all coming from the same place and wanting to head to the same place. Unlearning is universal because we've all been students of "learned deprivation." What's unique is how you get there.

Now we get to revisit and release the beliefs that aren't true. You can stop hiding the parts of yourself you think aren't worthy, strong, lovable, beautiful, or capable. You get to throw open the closet doors and let the skeletons out—they were never yours to begin with. We each have exactly what we need to walk our path. It is when we attempt to replicate someone else's journey that we find we're ill-equipped.

I thought I was doing everything I could to feel good because I was doing all the things. But I only had half the pieces of the puzzle. All the habits I'd developed until now revolved around how much I could give. But happiness is about our capacity to receive.

Throughout this book, I interchangeably use terms like happiness and joy to represent the common end goal we all seek. You may call it by a different name (wealthy, healthy, prestige, peaceful, fulfillment, etc.), but everything we strive for in life is done so because it's meant to make us feel good.

Happiness and joy have formal definitions, but they are also deeply personal to each of us. Before you proceed, I want you to take a moment to decide what those ideas look like for you. As you continue, know the words I chose are just placeholders for whatever makes you feel good.

Do you let yourself see all the love around you? Do you accept kind words? Do you offer them to yourself? Do you witness how far you've come? Or do you deprive yourself? Do you brush off your wins? Do you put yourself down? Offer to explain away a compliment? Do you see mostly what you aren't? High-vibe states put us in a frame of mind to receive from our life because it changes what we see in it. Happiness is like a message in a foggy mirror. It doesn't disappear when we feel down; we just haven't created the right conditions to see it.

Our default is to believe there's some lack within us. Nature has a role, but nurture plays a more significant role than you might realize. We are products of our environment. We see others living this low-vibe model, waiting for their true happiness to show up when. . . *the kids go to college, I retire, things slow down, the holidays are over.* You wait for that proverbial "when," only to shove happiness back down the list when something else asks for your attention. And trust me, something (or someone) *will* ask for it.

Feeling good is available to us at any moment if it's our habit to seek it. Habits can be defined as a "usual way of behaving." Way too often, we believe that the thing we call personality is set in stone, even if it's not helping us out. There's a blurry line between personality and habits. Engaging with the same behavior for so long makes it difficult to separate what we do from who we are. We forget that we can choose to change.

We are running on autopilot most of the time. But do you remember setting your course? The reason I'm asking is because whether we realize it or not, we have a trajectory set. But if we don't stop to question whether it still serves us, we might be blocking the very thing we're looking for: happiness.

When habits work for us, they create ease in our lives. When they don't, they put up barriers. And no matter how many times we go around them or over them, they pop back up in front of us. Until we replace them.

Take a good look around your life. Notice all the good things around you. Your habits helped make them possible. Take another look around at the things you'd like to get rid of or feel less of. Your habits also keep these things in your life. Good or bad, we tend to do the same things over and over. Most of us don't spend a lot of time focusing on what's working. You probably don't go around feeling extra good about yourself because you made it to work on time for the millionth day in a row or have a roof over your head. But we've all probably spent time regretting and feeling bad or guilty for the repetitive choices we'd rather not be making, like snapping at a loved one. Sometimes we make similar decisions so often we even believe that we're defective. *I'm bad with money. I always date the wrong guy. I never finish things. I'm always rushing.*

But you are not your choices. You can make new choices and have new habits. Offering ourselves new information is critical to our ability to make different decisions. If you keep putting yourself in the same situation, chances are that you'll end up making the same choices. The High Vibe Habits always offer us that new lens to see new possibilities within us and around us.

Okay, so we can agree that we have habits. We agree that it can be hard to distinguish between who we are (our nature) and what our habits are (nurture). I'm here to offer you five simple habits that will let you live less stressed so you can prioritize your health and happiness with consistency and without guilt. How do we bring in and create these new habits in our lives? The reason you're not doing what feels good or what's good for you probably isn't from lack of information. Almost everyone knows some part of what they "should" be doing: getting more sleep, eating fresh food, and moving their bodies.

I'll be the first to admit it, prioritizing yourself is hard. It means you are willing to pour time, money, and energy into something that is of little or no value to anyone else. Taking care of ourselves and letting ourselves feel good is simple. What's difficult are the beliefs we must possess to make the decisions that let us find space in our lives for ourselves. Destructive habits come from destructive beliefs.

To say no to life's constant requests is a stress-reducing act of well-being on its own. I'm not here to offer you a list of to-dos because, while feeling good is a universal desire, your specific path will be unique. There's certainly nothing wrong with doing things and creating healthy routines. But a huge part of my work is to help you first remove those stress habits that create obstacles in your life. Removing them opens us up to what's already in our lives without needing to create or do more. And when we do want to create new habits, we can do so with more ease. The High Vibe Habits are going to provide you with a supportive infrastructure. Here's the thing, if we don't change *how* we allocate our resources (time, money, and energy), we never have "enough" to make it to feeling good. We can't stay consistent enough to let joy, gratefulness, love, self-care, or connection become our habits.

It's such a reflex for us to think that doing more is the answer. So, instead of just listening to me, I invite you to reflect on your journey.

Have you ever written a gratefulness list? Do you remember how it made you feel? I love how connected and appreciative I feel for the people and things in my life. But in a few days, sometimes a few hours, the feeling starts to get diluted. One of my kids melts down, my computer glitches, or my husband snaps at me, and boom, I'm back to square one. Frustrated, stressed, and disconnected. You probably know people who seem super positive and always find something to be grateful for. And it's not because they're carrying a list around. Whether it was intentional or not, those people have been cultivating that habit.

Joy as a reflex. Sounds amazing, right? But if that's what's possible, what's happening right now? Where are your habits leading you? Most of us picked up our habits when we were young and still learning to navigate the world. We did the best we could and some of the skills we practiced have served us well. But over time, some begin to become a weight on our shoulders. Unlearning lets us reevaluate what is working for us and what's actually working against us and the life we want. It's a process of consciously and intentionally deciding what stays and what goes.

The work of unlearning is necessary to begin to permanently dismantle the walls we build that block us from our happiness, peace, and fulfillment. As children, we need others to create a safe space for us. As adults, we retrain ourselves to be that safe space for ourselves through unlearning. It doesn't mean we stop needing other people. It means we also get to learn how to give ourselves what we need: love, worthiness, and acceptance.

I'm adding a modern twist to Glinda's famous words, "You've always had the power dear; you just had to *un*learn it for yourself."

"

The fact that someone else loves you doesn't rescue you from the project of loving yourself.

—Sahaj Kohl

TWO

PERSPECTIVE

Once upon a time, there was a crustacean (let's just call it a shrimp). The little shrimp, born into the vast ocean, floats freely until finally, she lands herself a beautiful sea sponge to call home (it's called a Venus' flower basket if you're curious). A lucky fella lands on the same sponge, and they stake their claim, together making it their permanent residence. The sponge offers the shrimp food, protection, and shelter. The shrimp offer the sponge good hygiene. A perfect symbiotic match. Everything they need is here—paradise.

Or is it?

Things are rarely what they seem. Darkness lurks, and it's not just from the lack of light. Like all creatures, these shrimps are growing. Nothing out of the ordinary there. Except the delicate lace pattern of the Venus' flower basket doesn't grow at the same pace.

By adulthood, these shrimps allow themselves to be trapped, forever. The small cutouts that once kept predators at bay now hold them hostage. The trade seems to suit them fine, but it got me thinking.

Before you go judging the little shrimps, take a look at your life. We don't stray too far from those crustaceans' lives. We all do this type of barter at some point. We give up our joy, our voice, our opinions, and even our strengths to appease people, fit in, and get praise. What freedoms have you traded for safety and connection? I've held back my feelings to make room for someone else's. I handed over my happiness to avoid confrontation. I know others who've given up their dreams or the love of their life to feel accepted by their families. It's time to recognize that we pick up beliefs and develop the habits that stem from them perpetuating a dangerous (and false) idea— that happiness is fragile.

The Problem

Experiencing happiness is natural. It doesn't require as much as we think it does. When it doesn't show up for us, we might be

44

tempted to believe in the myth that it's elusive and exclusive. But for joy to become our reflex, we get to give up the belief that someone (or something) else can give it to us. This (learned) belief is what directs us to erect barriers to our happiness. You don't need to spend your energy "creating" or "finding" happiness. Sunshine, hugs, rain, a walk—happiness is everywhere. Somewhere along the way to adulthood, we stop believing in this kind of simplicity, but the truth is simple. You can experience happiness when you allow it in, in other words, when you stop working against it.

I want to get clear on what these self-made obstacles look like, sound like, and feel like because they aren't abstract ideas. They are very real habits that change the way we show up every single day. There are a lot of obstacles in the world created by family, culture, and society, but battling those often begins from a deeply personal place. The High Vibe Habits do create changes in our outer world, but they do so because they change our internal landscape. Let's get curious (that's a High Vibe Habit!) so we can get clarity (another habit!) and start to recognize them in our own lives. We have to find them before we can deconstruct them.

We are all products of our environment, where rings of pressure (our family, culture, and society) have brought us up to practice what I call "learned deprivation." These are skills that were essential to our survival that we now rely on too heavily, making them more of a hindrance than a help.

Whether your habits are distracting or have swung all the way to destructive, learned deprivation relies heavily on the idea that feeling bad is normal or even good. Feeling poorly is supposed to motivate us. And it does, sort of. Many people find traditional success with this original model. (But not necessarily happiness, peace, or fulfillment.) In the "do more" fallacy, it's the *only* way to motivate ourselves and sometimes the only way to communicate with ourselves. We learn to condemn parts of ourselves for not being "enough."

These beliefs can come from us, but they can also come from others. Either way, their origin can become indistinguishable because we often shift from audience to author. Everything we hear, see, and experience is filtered through our minds and becomes a part of us. We tell ourselves what we aren't, long after our parents, teachers, or peers do. We infer all sorts of things year after year and can end up with a distorted view of ourselves and the world. The beliefs we hold onto as adults, the ones we use to navigate the world, were decided by a kid—our childhood self. How often do we stop to ask ourselves if those words are true or support us? And how much time, energy, and money do we pour into the decisions we make based on those thoughts?

Energy has always been a precious resource, and our brains evolved to be as efficient as possible to conserve it. Categorization is one of those efficiency methods[4]. It's why we create meaning out of information so quickly. This is helpful in many ways, but not so much when it comes to understanding or changing our beliefs. Everything that passes through us gets assigned meaning and value. But the truth is that before we get our hands on them, all events are neutral. Have you ever

---

[4] Brinson, Sam. *"Why We Divide Ourselves—Categorical Thinking and a Lazy Brain."* Sam Brinson, May 11, 2017. https://www.sambrinson.com/categorical-thinking/.

experienced a snowstorm? Was it good or bad? As an adult who has to shovel the driveway and get to work, you might think it's unfortunate. But when you were a kid, snow days were the best thing ever. Every event, like a delayed flight or getting lost, can be seen from many angles at any time. We choose to believe if it's good or bad and can train our minds to reframe situations.

How does this work against us? We are quietly fed a set of virtues and vices. Our thoughts are shaped by these environmental influences. Some of these are positive and help support a healthy, thriving community, while others are like poison. *Be good. Be quiet. Be nice.* As blanket statements, these are easily interpreted to discourage boundaries, opinions, and confidence thanks to our quick neural processing.

Remember, thoughts that remain within us create our belief system. Those beliefs affect every decision, interaction, choice, thought, and dream you have about yourself and the world. Judgment, guilt, shame, regret, and comparison are invisible forces of learned deprivation that can quickly turn into very real, very visible hurdles and hardships that we work to overcome. They manifest as lower incomes, health problems, sadness, unhealthy relationships, regret, stress, and burnout.

A big part of learned deprivation is the labeling process that teaches us to see ourselves, others, and the world in terms of good and bad. There are agreed-upon characteristics (often dependent on gender, culture, and family) that are considered better—like extraversion and assertiveness— which means there are others that we should consider not so great. By labeling our emotions, thoughts, and behaviors in these black-and-white terms, we tend to demonize parts of ourselves. We try to cover up or make up for this innate "lack" we believe we have. And this feels especially bad when it conflicts with our true nature.

Having access to a wide range of emotions doesn't mean there's something wrong with you. It means you're human. None of what I share is about fixing you. There's nothing wrong with you. You've just been practicing some habits that might not be serving you. The High Vibe Habits let you find balance within by increasing your capacity to receive (information, kindness, rest) and access constructive tools for a more objective perspective.

HIGH VIBE REFRAME

EMOTIONS = INFORMATION

Having a full range of emotions and feelings is healthy but so is knowing how to harvest what they're telling you so you can move on healthily. Supportive and constructive—that's the High Vibe way.

Part of identifying High Vibe is figuring out what a low vibe is. Where are our current habits taking us? And what are they actually doing to us? I promised you real examples because it's the fastest, easiest, and surest way to understand low vibe living. My journey has uncovered some surprising beliefs I didn't even realize I held. Some of the seemingly ordinary childhood moments, which were originally filed away as nothing, actually ended up being the beginning of beliefs that had me heading for a life of empty instead of full.

I learned early on that others would give me things: praise, confidence, adoration, and pride. Things I hadn't yet figured out I could give to myself.

I earned my first penny at four years old. I was sitting in the backseat of my mom's gray Honda, running my hand over the fuzzy gray fabric, warm from the sun. Red, green, blue, and yellow, a guilty reminder of the Fantastic Sam's crayons I once left in the backseat of my mother's beloved Honda that didn't survive the summer sun. A bump in the road brought me back as we pulled off Thirty-Second Street; I looked up. I was staring at the orange, all-caps letters of the car wash when my brother turned to me.

"Can you read that?" He asked.

I paused and confirmed, "Automatic."

My brother fished out a penny from the little nook of the door handle and handed it to me. His smile told me everything. He was proud of me. And it meant the world to me. He was the sun, and I was basking in his rays.

I grew up with him always cheering me on. His adoration meant the world to me. But later, I realized, it would have a string attached. He could pull it and take it back just as quickly. This wasn't unique to my brother. Anyone can if we give them that power. When people's words have the power to lift us, they also have the power to weigh us down. What someone else gives us, they can take away. What we offer ourselves is forever. The energy of seeking and proving is very different than the confident energy of knowing who we are and what we are worth.

For decades that "seeking" shaped my behavior because I was afraid of losing any label I wanted to be identified with. I liked feeling special. Who doesn't? Especially because I didn't necessarily think I was. My brother's adoration felt like a gift I couldn't find on my own. Someone else's beliefs feel more powerful than our own when we haven't decided for ourselves what is true.

This feeling of not being enough became a part of the way I operated until I found a constructive alternative. I utilized deprivation as a part of my motivational drive. Not feeling good was not only familiar, but I also depended on it as a guiding force. I think a lot of us do. The feeling of pushing myself hard, becoming exhausted, and finding something I could've done better is what I believed fed my drive and therefore my success. A part of me was afraid that if I felt good I might get complacent. The truth is that seeking external validation not only doesn't feel good, but it's a never-ending cycle. There's no stickiness in what we receive and what we earn. The praise, the proof, and the satisfaction of reaching a goal slip right through our fingers. No celebrations allowed. We're just left asking ourselves, what's next?

You can fill in the blank as it relates to your life. Who do you feel holds the answer for you? A man? A job? An address? A car? A family? A salary?

The unpredictable nature of happiness comes from being primarily influenced by things outside of yourself. All the old distracting habits say we don't get to give ourselves what we need. They tell us to look around us for love and acceptance and outside for proof of our worthiness, value, intelligence, and success. The fleeting nature of happiness exists because we're waiting for someone or something to offer it to us. That's the distorted vision we develop through the habits of learned deprivation. The High Vibe Habits are like corrective lenses that let us see that we get to offer ourselves what we need.

The High Vibe Habits aren't for fixing, they're for transforming. They're here to refocus your attention from the distraction of pain from low-vibe feelings to the constructive possibilities that come with feeling good. The old habits of learned deprivation rely on motivation through suffering. But dwelling in pain is distracting at best (like mild stress) and destructive at worst (like substance abuse and chronic disease). The main habits of this old model are comparison, judgment, guilt, shame, and regret. Growing up and living in this environment means we grow up steeped in this line of thought. They make us feel alone, lacking, and unworthy. These feelings and habits can be passed down even in a loving home because they aren't passed down to purposely harm us. They are passed down by habit and beliefs.

I'd been blessed with a loving family full of larger-than-life personalities. Being the youngest in a multigenerational household, I'd always felt like I'd grown up amongst giants. Their character traits and successes would become the notches against which I would measure myself. And I often fell short. In my eyes, they were smart, strong, beloved, accomplished, and fearless. I wanted to find my place among them and to be worthy of the love and adoration they gave me.

If the nut doesn't fall far from the tree, I'd always felt like I'd been swept up in a tornado and deposited far, far away. Because as a kid, I felt nothing like my family, but I wanted nothing more than to be like my family. I didn't realize and couldn't see many of my strengths because I was looking to replicate what I saw around me. I thought that being my family's equal meant I needed to be the same, a version of them. I wanted to move through the world with the same ease I saw them exhibit. They had confidence, authority, charm, intelligence, and courage. I wasn't sure I recognized those things in me. And slowly, I stopped noticing what I was because I couldn't stop noticing what I wasn't.

Comparison is always relative. Childhood usually exposes us to the same few groups of people. It's in this small world that we first find our place and ourselves. But where we lie on any spectrum depends on those around us. Everyone has strengths, but if we're looking for the same ones, we overlook and undervalue our own because they are different. We see ourselves as fixed and begin to live that story. Comments, teachings, and praise delineate desired characteristics that we attempt to embody. And they create feelings of lack when we fall short of those ideals. It's reinforced in our everyday language: *I am, I can't, I don't.* It comes from others: *you can't, she isn't, and you'll never.* Phrases like that hold us back when they separate us from what we would like to be, do, and have. We use them on ourselves and other people, whether we are putting them on a pedestal or cutting them down. Growing up, I found myself using these as I observed the traits my family had.

I never finish things. I always pick the wrong men. I never say the right thing. How many of these "I knew it" moments do you have? The "See! I told you!" kind that proves to you that you aren't something. Lack is painful and pain is distracting. Avoiding it becomes our motivation, our payoff. If I keep being the same me, I know what to expect. When I choose to be or do something different, I break away from expectations (my own and other people's). Getting out of our comfort zone is how we grow, but it's also where we feel vulnerable.

Remember, learned deprivation is about taking natural tendencies and overusing them in ways that don't support us. Confirmation bias is one of those. It's the tendency we all have to prove ourselves right (regardless of whether it's beneficial). Our brains search for evidence that supports our current beliefs and ideas (even more so when there's an emotional connection to the belief)[5]. I've heard women share stories where they were told they were ugly, dumb, difficult, incapable, worthless, or unworthy of love. Those women refused to let that stop them from going out into the world, but a seed was planted. And confirmation bias nurtured it. If we believe we are unworthy, the world will keep supplying us with that evidence even if we don't want it to be true. Our beliefs can be self-fulfilling prophecies, creating the realities we most fear. Where our thoughts go, energy flows. Are you focused on what you aren't? Or what you are or would like to be? With intention, confirmation bias can also support us.

---

[5] Simkus, Julia. Updated June 22, 2023. *Confirmation Bias In Psychology: Definition & Examples.* Simply Psychology. https://www.simplypsychology.org/confirmation-bias.html

As visual learners, we are always observing what's acceptable and what's not. We learn to fear the consequences of making different choices when we're young because we are dependent on others for our survival. In his book *Resilient*, Rick Hanson talks about how our brain's job is to learn how to make sure our basic needs (safety, satisfaction, and connection) are met. This isn't all bad. It can work *for* us. When we understand our nature, we can know what thoughts to nurture.

Without arming ourselves with that strategy, it's easy to notice that we get judged, categorized, and labeled, quickly. We hear people talking about us, others, and themselves. We grow up learning to please, contort, shrink, or expand so we feel accepted, loved, and safe.

In preschool, my teachers had me take some sort of placement test and deemed me worthy of skipping ahead. I left my glue-eating peers behind and found myself at the tail end of kindergarten as the youngest in my class. I'm not sure I had any idea what this meant, but I had been labeled smart, and it felt good.

A few years later, I tested into our school's gifted program, where I had already begun to feel enormous pressure to keep up and prove I belonged. Fear of failure began to take up a lot of space in me. My very intelligent older brother had been pointing out to me for some time that we may both be smart but not be fooled that we were the same. It was typical sibling banter, but it left an impression on me.

Then, in my fifth-grade year, we moved. I had to retest into the gifted program in our new town. I was so nervous. I had been able to keep up with the other gifted students in my class before, but a test? Yikes. To my great relief, I passed and was enrolled in the new gifted program. Whew.

That victory was short-lived. My brother confided in me that he had some secret information. I hadn't passed the test, he said. But the councilors had agreed with my parents to let me in since I'd already been in a gifted program. I felt crushed. Shattered. Did they feel sorry for me? Did they think I couldn't cut it? I knew it, I thought. I wasn't a good test taker and now I knew why—I wasn't that smart. I'd probably just been lucky the first time around. (Decades later I'd find out it was a lie, and I had passed the test.)

Determined but scared, I decided to prove to all of them, especially my brother, that I was good enough. I was smart, I kept telling myself while ignoring the other voices that said otherwise. But I would go through the rest of my academic days feeling like a free diver, painfully holding my breath until I received my grade or scores, exhaling with relief that, so far, I was keeping up the charade.

Adoration is tricky, as it can turn into imitation. But when we try to duplicate anyone, we run the risk of feeling insecure. Which makes sense if you think about it. We have to try to be someone else. Being ourselves comes naturally.

Rather than being able to celebrate the differences between my family and my peers, I strove to be the same. I confused the same for equal when the truth is we already have what we need. We are each born enough. It is when we attempt to replicate someone else's journey that we find we're ill-equipped.

That's where the unlearning comes into play. We get to stop and question all the beliefs and thoughts that don't let us feel good. The things we tell ourselves that don't let us celebrate, rest, relax, and love ourselves. As we got older, my brother would complement my unique intelligence and ability to create success in many disciplines. Words of affirmation are nice, but if they are a "new" concept they might be at odds with our preexisting identity. Youth is when we formulate certainty in who we are, not realizing that we might misjudge ourselves. We would never let a child run a business or our lives, yet as adults, we go through the world based on a child's (our inner child's) beliefs of who we are and what we are capable of. But we always have the opportunity to evolve if we intentionally offer ourselves the self-compassion and patience to unlearn old stories.

It took me decades, and honestly, motherhood, before I was willing to untangle my past. I think it's easier to be brave for someone else. I found a tremendous well of courage in a role where I am always advocating, supporting, teaching, and protecting. I was willing to do for my children what I couldn't fully commit to on my own — rewrite my story. To decide for myself what stays and what goes. To have the hard conversations. To sit with discomfort and pain. To have an evolving vision and enjoy the journey. To shed decades' worth of expectations to lead by example. To show my children, myself, and other women how powerful we each can be. It's not until we're ready and willing to initiate change that we stop imitating and start embracing the power in our uniqueness.

Once we get so focused on what we lack, it's easy to see how we start working to overcome, or hide, the parts of ourselves that don't fit in. We begin to sacrifice what makes us, us. It's an easy habit because we're already wired for it.

Negativity is very real and can be a very active part of our mental processing. All of us have this tendency to remember more of the bad stuff *and* file it away as important. It's called a negativity bias or positive-negative asymmetry[6]. Just wait, it gets better (or maybe I should say worse). In addition to focusing on these unpleasantries, we revisit them! Over and over again thanks to negative

[6] Kendra Cherry. *"What Is the Negativity Bias?"* Verywell Mind, November 13, 2023. https://www.verywellmind.com/negative-bias-4589618

rumination, which only connects us more deeply with the negative belief[7]. This Ice-Age-old inclination toward negative experiences that originally developed to keep us alive contributes significantly to our present-day struggles. So, rest easy. You're not the only one who finds the good things in life so slippery.

For years, I believed the path to success, pride, admiration, and fulfillment would lie in my ability to overcome who I was. It would be decades before I allowed myself to not only believe that I was enough but to realize the power within could only be unleashed when I could completely be myself. If we keep focusing on what we're not, we'll never be able to be the best of what we are.

Women as a whole believe in our ability to give, do, and go the extra mile. I was never afraid of hard work. Discipline came easily to me so I made a plan: I would use my observation skills to watch for excellence, then learn how to emulate it. I would pick and choose all the traits I wanted. Square by

---

[7] Hanson, Rick. *Resilient: How to Grow an Unshakable Core of Calm, Strength, and Happiness,* 2018, 44.
https://www.amazon.com/Resilient-Grow-Unshakable-Strength-Happiness/dp/0451498844

square, like a patchwork quilt, I would come together as a masterpiece. It's how I would make myself and my family proud. I practiced this in my teens, twenties, and even my thirties. All the habits I was developing were around giving. I learned to pour all of myself into whatever was in front of me. I saw all the women in my life doing this. Society says success is created by our capacity to give. But our health, happiness, and continued success is created by the additional ability to receive. That's the one no one teaches us.

My work quickly became my worth. Life was a performance. According to my grades, achievements, titles, accolades, degrees, and job titles, people believed I was doing everything right. But everything didn't *feel* right.

I lived somewhere between the fear of failure and the stress of succeeding. It's easy to believe anxiety and worry are only a problem when they're crippling or when they stop us. But I expended enormous amounts of energy managing my mental anxieties—all the '*I should be's*'. I think deep down I knew I was more powerful than I felt, but you don't really benefit from kind of believing in yourself. That's the most self-sabotaging type of belief. You put yourself out on a limb, but the weight of your fears all but ensures you can't take flight.

The truth is we forget that if we are great at any moment, that's a sign of what lies within us at *every* moment. Uncovering these happiness barriers means accepting the truth. Believing in yourself is an all-or-nothing game. There are moments when we feel brilliant. And the moments we fall short aren't proof we are frauds, but proof we are human. They aren't reasons to stop believing, they are opportunities to learn how to support ourselves. It's tiring constantly proving to the world what you are. That lifestyle keeps you chasing that carrot that's always just out of reach.

What does it take for you to feel enough?

That lifestyle choice led me to feel like I had to earn anything that felt good. But you don't need to earn happiness, love, joy, peace, or worthiness. It's in believing that you just get to have these things that you can offer the world your greatest contribution— your true self.

What happens when we don't accept that truth? We give. And give. And give. Hoping that our partner, parents, children, and friends will give enough back to us to keep us going and feeling good. That expectation leads to disappointment. I invite you to take on a new perspective: I get to take care of myself. And you get to take care of yourself. And that's not scary or sad. That's freedom. It means what we seek from life is only partially accomplished through giving. The balance that most of us work so hard to achieve comes from improving our ability to receive.

Learned deprivation plants many seeds within us. One is the belief that if we aren't giving, we might be taking. It makes us feel guilty for using time for pleasure, rest, or self-care. And it's based on the promise that someone else will give me what I need. But you don't have to place such a heavy burden on your relationships, and you don't have to wait around for anyone else before you get what you need in life.

We've covered a few brain presets that might currently be overactive and lead to thoughts that distract us from our goal of enjoying life. But we don't need to or want to, get rid of them completely. We just want to stop overusing them. All of these built-in mechanisms help us survive. And we get to learn how to remaster them so that we can thrive. All emotions are information[8]. Have you ever thought about your feelings like that? Information? We think and then feel something as an experience that is filtered through our mind and gets assigned meaning. The thoughts we have and the feelings we feel are all intended to guide us in our decision-making process.

But we even manage to have emotions about our emotions. That's a never-ending judgment loop until we become whatever it is we believe we're supposed to be. *Quiet. Nice. Less sensitive. Tough-skinned.*

Feelings, especially for women, are used as a weapon against us. The truth? Emotions and feelings are information. No more, no less. They allow us to gain access to knowledge that would otherwise be lost. The mind-body connection, often seen as a spiritual concept, plays a crucial role in our lives. You can get lost in the intricacies of emotions and feelings, but the important takeaway is this: Feelings and emotions alter our state of being and influence our mental

---

[8] Davis, Tchiki. The Berkeley Well-Being Institute. *"Emotion: Definition, Theories, & Examples,"* n.d. https://www.berkeleywellbeing.com/emotion.html

and physiological states. The signals they send alter our chemical state on a cellular level, affecting our ability to learn, problem-solve, and recall memories, to name a few[9]. Why does the Superman pose work so effectively? Altering our posture sends chemical signals to our brains, which alter our emotional state as well. Take a minute to think about your own experiences. What are you thinking? How do you feel?

I've shared some of the science behind our habits, but you "get it" because you've experienced it. A fearful thought that ties your stomach in knots. An excited one that gives you butterflies. The mind and body are a two-way communication system designed to work together—a strength. But only if we utilize the information. Emotions and feelings are the messengers of our belief system.

---

[9] Tyng, Chai M., Hafeez U. Amin, Mohamad N. M. Saad, and Aamir S. Malik. *"The Influences of Emotion on Learning and Memory."* Frontiers in Psychology 8 (August 24, 2017) https://www.frontiersin.org/journals/psychology/articles/10.3389/fpsyg.2017.01454/full

The Solution

There are only three places we can be: the past, present, or future. Not literally, of course, but they're the only spaces our minds can occupy. The High Vibe Habits are designed to prepare you for wherever you find yourself. In the coming chapters, we'll dive into exactly how each of the five C's can support you, but for now, let's zoom out and figure out how we can begin to access them in the first place.

Before you can choose something new, you've got to know what you want to change or that you're making a less desirable choice in the first place. Awareness is the first step. The essence of what I'm saying boils down to this: I must recognize when I'm experiencing a low-vibe feeling. Then I've got to offer myself a way up and out into a higher vibrational emotion. To get rid of a habit, you need to replace it. Microdosing happiness is that bridge. It's as simple as:

Step 1: Ask yourself, how am I feeling?

Step 2: Then ask, what could I do to help myself feel better?

It's a pause, a pattern interrupter, allowing you to take back control and get intentional about being the solution. If you're questioning your emotional state, you're giving yourself a chance to choose your own experience. Imagine a container of water and two bottles of ink, one gray and one blue. If we are the water, the choices we make lead us to feel bad (gray ink) or feel good (blue ink). We are altered drop by drop (choice by choice) to become either predominantly gray or blue. Microdosing happiness is this drop-by-drop process of intentionally choosing the blue ink. A small decision chosen over and over again creates a big impact.

Any of us can remember one thing. That's why I'm just going to ask you to focus on this one simple question: *How do I feel?* And let that one question be the doorway to your new habits. The more you practice the more in tune you'll be with yourself. You'll be amazed at how quickly you can begin to recognize feeling misaligned.

I didn't realize how much time I spent feeling poorly or low until I prioritized feeling good. The same goes for most of the women I've worked with. It's easy for the doer to get things done, check off their list, or come up with new things to add to that list. What's challenging is figuring out how to let themselves rest, pause, and take care of themselves without guilt.

How can one question transform your life? Because by asking yourself the question, *how do I feel*, you're reminding yourself that the answer matters. *You matter.* And that you get to be the one to make sure you keep feeling good. Does this mean you'll always feel on top of the world? No. But hitting the pause button gives you the chance to *respond* instead of react. It's what opens the door for you to choose a High Vibe Habit instead of a distracted habit that keeps you feeling stuck and low.

I mentioned earlier that the effects of a distracted lifestyle aren't abstract. They lead us to make choices with very real consequences. The very essence of how we are taught to give is by giving more than we have. It's another situation where you are only winning when you're losing. Depletion isn't a long-term strategy and yet, so many of us build lives on this unsustainable, always-on model.

We wake up one day with a spouse, children, and so much work (career, caregiving, or otherwise). With all these roles, we begin to forget who we were before them and who we are with them. We find ourselves in a yes-culture, where we cram more and more into our lives until the only things we're not saying "yes" to are the things that we want. We're overworked and that leads us to feel underwhelmed with our life. Ever wondered, *is this all there is?* We plan and wait for the chance to break free: a weekend, a vacation, or even retirement.

The same old strategies seem to be failing you. You blame yourself. You're not as focused because you have a family now. You're low on energy because you're taking on more and more to prove to everyone that you're capable of doing it all. You're supposed to look good all the time, be at home, go to work, follow your ambitions, and make it all look easy. Everyone else does, right? So, when did it all stop working?

You probably find yourself hearing everyone else tell you how they went through what you're going through and that's just how things are. And that only feels worse because now you feel bad that you feel bad. It's a vicious cycle that leads us to a low-vibe state. Doing something different takes practice and very few of us have the example set for us.

Without a sustainable giving strategy, burnout happens. Working harder isn't always the solution. Life is a long game and without a long-term plan, sacrifice becomes a lifestyle instead of a stage. We all want to give, but the irony is that we have to learn how to receive if we want to keep giving.

I know you're important. You're worth taking time for. You deserve health and happiness as much as the next person. But when you don't prioritize yourself or your needs, even the best-case scenarios can hold dark surprises.

So, what happens when you don't ask yourself how you feel? Why you want to ask yourself that question is important because of what happens when you don't.

Rewinding about twenty years, I can clearly see all of these self-oppressive mechanisms in action. In my mid-twenties, I landed my dream job. Working at a luxury Italian fashion house was a seriously pinch-me moment. Until it wasn't. The reality was much different than the dream. Getting to tell people about what I did and where I worked felt like the validation I had worked hard for. The proof that I was good enough. There are only a handful of these positions spread across a few companies—and I held one.

But in the end, the excitement of sharing my title was not enough to carry me through the hellish days. I tried my best to show up, perform, and exceed expectations. The only problem was that I wasn't the problem. (This in no way implies I was perfect, only that no one deserves to be treated poorly.) Anyone who has experienced a toxic work environment understands this. My boss, for reasons unknown, didn't respect me, and she wasn't afraid to show it.

This blew my mind. Not only had we worked together in the past, but she actually recruited me for this position. Deciding to accept the position was one of the most emotionally difficult choices I had made. I left a job I loved for the promise of one that I expected to love. It made the toxic experience doubly painful. I was yelled at, given the work of several people, and harassed. The emotional abuse was cringeworthy. Every time my office phone would ring, new knots would form in my stomach. Even my office mates would wince with the ringing. I had never experienced anything like this. She was relentless. And me? I just kept on trying to meet her expectations.

Working long hours in New York City is nothing to write home about. But being the only person working five-plus hours more than everyone in your office? That was. I waited in front of the building at 6 a.m. sharp for the doorman to unlock the front door. I left through the freight elevator at 11 p.m. because the main elevator and building entrance were locked. I exited the building the same way the trash did—out the back.

Traveling to Milan for Fashion Week turned into a special kind of nightmare. I worked around the clock. The lights in the building went off around eleven at night. I continued to work using a desk lamp. I sat in the dull yellow spotlight, eating my vending machine "dinner," waiting to be swallowed by the darkness around me. While the rest of my team was fine dining in Milan, I scrounged for coins for the finicky vending machine hoping it would spit out something to assuage my hunger. The machine and I both went hungry the following night when I was stuck with only bills and no change. And that's the good part of the nightmare.

One night, I went to bed exhausted (nothing unusual there). But I woke up the next morning feeling a bit more like myself, refreshed. The smile that began appearing on my face never quite made it to fruition. There could be only one reason that I felt this good—I overslept. I tore out of my room and, of course, ran into my boss in the lobby. Her glare instantly shrunk my five-foot-seven-inch frame into a mouse's. Her eyes said it all, *I better have everything ready for her, or else*. I feared what the "or else" would be.

The only saving grace was the kindness of a coworker (the tech guy) that came with us. His company and kindness in those dark days were the only things holding me together. I made it back home, physically, but I felt like a shell of myself.

The crazy part is that I never complained—not once—during my whole time working there. I thought for sure I could prove to my boss that I could do it all and to her liking. I wanted to prove to myself, too, that I could somehow be enough. Looking back, I can see it was never about me. But back then, in the thick of things, I did what any proud achiever would do. I worked harder.

Working hard was the only choice I saw available to me. I would reach a breaking point, and even when resigning seemed like the only way out, I kept going. In the end, it was someone else's kindness that offered me what I needed. The vice president of the company came to my office one night to check in on me. He said that another director had wanted to bring my situation to his attention. Many people believed I was being treated poorly. Those words brought me to tears. To know that it wasn't all in my head, that it wasn't all my fault, was an enormous relief. If it weren't for those kind souls, I wonder how much more I would've endured. I did resign shortly after, but I left with a little piece of me feeling like it was my fault. Maybe I had failed.

The anxiety has faded but the memories have not. I see so many places where I could've found ways to support myself. But I didn't have access to the same tools I use today. I turned away from all the facts that pointed to my capacity to succeed and grow and leaned into the fear of not being good enough. Those unproductive thoughts led to so much misaligned action. What I wanted was to flourish in this position, but what I allowed myself to do was be squashed.

How does this happen? I had a good sense that I was not feeling good about myself or my work environment. I asked that first question (*how am I feeling?*), but I didn't value the answer. I didn't know what to do with my feelings about this experience. That incoming information seemed irrelevant. So, I shoved it down, I cried, and I felt bitter. I wanted this thing that I'd worked so hard for. And now that I had it, not flourishing in it felt like failing.

It's so easy to get lost somewhere between our fear of failure and the stress of success because we spend our energy trying to show the world that we're enough. And when our energy is spent trying to figure out how to be enough for someone else, we miss the chance to shine as who we already are. Does this mean that you shouldn't keep learning and growing? No. But it does mean that sometimes things in life aren't a great fit, no matter how hard you try. But a poor fit isn't a failure, it's knowledge.

We find what we seek. And by that, I mean we find what our subconscious seeks. Where your attention goes, energy flows. Our mission is not to survive in any condition but to find one where we can thrive. Later on, one of my coaches would give me some great advice: "Just because you can, doesn't mean you should." I took that dream job because it sounded fun, and prestigious, and would prove that I had made it. Sometimes other people's opinions become a form of compensation more valuable than a salary or our feelings. I was willing to be unhappy because I thought it was worth it. If this was what success looked like, I was learning to deal with what it felt like. That type of compass takes us where someone else chooses, not where we want to be.

It makes sense that as children we're looking to find a safe space within our family and culture. But as adults, it's important to transition into *being* that safe space for ourselves. When we shift our beliefs, we change our thoughts and take aligned action. We make a healthy vision possible through our habits. And evolving that vision isn't a failure, it's growth.

Brain science keeps reminding us that we make better decisions when we work from a constructive place because we're actually using a different part of the brain. Living and working in fear, real or perceived, closes off access to these parts. You can reduce the amount of resistance in your life, personally and professionally, by simply changing the way you think. Like a domino effect, new thoughts trigger new actions which lead to new outcomes. And in every one of those scenarios, you get to be in control of yourself.

Distracted living deceives many of us because, whether it's distracting or destructive, many aspects of it are praised by others. Self-sacrifice, overworking, busyness, and exhaustion are worn as badges of honor, displaying how "dedicated" we are to our lives and work. Don't worry about how often you get distracted and start getting intentional about choosing a constructive habit. What's possible is a life of physical and mental prosperity.

You're either making a distracted or constructive choice and they feel, sound, and look very different. You may not be used to arming yourself with the knowledge of feeling, but it's the easiest way to identify how you're living your life. This is *not* another way for you to judge or compare yourself. Think of this as a map. "You are here," it's that dot you look for when you walk into a new mall or park. Before you begin any journey, you need to get your bearings. Then you can ask, *where would I like to be?*

Feelings can seem vague, but there are actually a lot of cues our bodies send us to let us know which direction we're heading. Just identifying the feelings will help you be more in tune with what to look out for and make you better at catching yourself early on if you're headed downward.

Check out this chart.

Distracted	Constructive
> constriction	> expansion
> resistance/fight	> ease/flow
> exhaustion/defense	> progress/offense
> cutting down	> building up
> reactive	> responsive
> problem	> solution

VS

Chart I - These are the different emotional or physical sensations that accompany either a distracted mind or a constructive one.

Which side of the line are you on right now?

With each choice (thought or action), you head in one direction or the other.

Distracted habits trigger several feelings, thoughts, and sensations that generally lead to more stress because they focus on the problem at hand, or our lack, or leave us feeling like a victim. All these are valid, but not very productive.

Distracted living feels constrictive, both literally and figuratively. Physically, you exhibit shallow breathing and tense muscles. Mentally, your thoughts are constricted by doubt or fear. Indecision might be a problem. Your focus is primarily on controlling the outcome, instead of focusing on the process. It's totally normal to anticipate or hope for a specific end goal, but when there is fear around other people's expectations, you may not be optimizing your brain's full potential. You're problem oriented. You "what if" worst-case possibilities or decide you just know what's going to happen. Your spouse leaves town for work and your thoughts home in on how difficult it's going to be to manage the kids' school, meals, and activities, plus your elderly dog. Your anxiety builds with your anticipation of difficulty and disaster, rather than just managing what happens.

Wondering if deprivation might be your form of motivation? Do you make yourself earn everything? Coffee? Free time? Maybe even kind words? You're sure if you don't beat yourself up, you won't do better next time. Gratefulness might feel like your ceiling. It limits your success by not feeling like you can ask for more or maybe that you even deserve more. There's often a feeling of juggling many things without a feeling of progress like you're playing defense. You feel like you're the only one who can get things done the way you want them, the way they should be done. You're the only one who can meet your expectations.

Just as learned deprivation and distracted behaviors cause our minds and bodies to respond with constriction, a high-vibrational state (constructive behavior) does the opposite. Expansion is the reflex when we feel good. We're physically and mentally more limber. Our posture is more open and upright. Think about how the Superman pose works on our psyche. In this exercise, you're using your body to send signals to your brain. You feel more confident, relaxed, and capable. When problems arise, you see solutions with more ease and are thoughtful and more responsive instead of reactive. You have more pat-yourself-on-the-back moments because you allow yourself to witness your progress, growth, and wins. This gives you the energy to get even more done.

Think about the last really good day you had. It's not that bad things didn't happen; you just weren't focused on them. You probably got more done without feeling any more exhausted by it. You might even have felt really proud of yourself for the way you maneuvered through your day and its challenges. You might have even found the time to tackle something you've been meaning to get to. I bet you were even nicer to people and went out of your way for someone else. All this and more is what happens when we feel good. Making space for our needs naturally makes us more available to serve, do, and give.

There's no judgment for being on one side or the other. I want you to use this as a diagnostic tool. Do you utilize or feel one or more of these distracted elements consistently? The High Vibe Habits aren't a guarantee that you'll never lose your focus again. They're a path back to the clarity, control, and confidence you need to live the life you want. And microdosing happiness will be your North Star leading you back to that constructive path of being, doing, and living. Distracted living doesn't feel good for any of us because of the stress it creates. You can't be low vibe and high vibe at the same time. Staying stuck in low-vibrational states creates chronic stress.

Chronic stress has become so common that we forget that treating it isn't the only option. Being reactive is one choice, but being proactive is another. We can develop habits that help us avoid it (chronic stress, not all stress) in the first place. What's the cost of the reactive mindset?

Oppressive mental environments take a physical toll on us. Stress and burnout are rampant and major contributors to the conditions that rob us of quality of life at the least and quantity of life at the worst. All this disease is becoming normalized and demoralizes us further as we focus on how the body and mind go wrong.

Inevitably utilizing distracted tools leads to "empty," whether it's in one area (relationships, career, finances) or the whole thing. While it can produce success, it gradually shifts our focus to fear: the fear of losing what we have. Maintaining a lifestyle or an image can cost dollars, health, and happiness.

But it is possible for more to go right. Instead of feeling the urgency to squeeze more and more in, we can feel more empowered by learning how to squeeze more out of life. We can embrace the idea that there is enough time to do what matters when we know how.

Five habits simplify your life so you're able to create the energy, time, motivation, and plan that fit your life and lead to *your* happiness. For some people that looks like more time at work, for some, it'll be less. For some it's starting a business, for others it's retiring. Unlearning lets you redefine terms and the High Vibe Habits are your guardrails that keep you on track and moving forward.

There are probably things you'd tell your younger self if you could. Words of wisdom that you've earned along the way. But your journey isn't over yet. Aligning your vision and your actions reduces the regret of what you know you want to avoid. I know that simple doesn't mean easy. That's why this whole High Vibe transformation is built on taking the smallest steps with consistency.

Let's be done scaling, hurdling, and maneuvering around self-made obstacles. Let's make new mistakes instead of the same ones over and over again. Progress is more gratifying and motivating than we realize. Your "best" is more powerful than perfection. But know it will fluctuate depending on your internal state. Commit to what it takes to keep yourself in the highest vibrational state possible and see how the other pieces fall into place. No more demonizing parts of yourself. Bring it all into perspective as information. You can allow yourself to decide what you want and who you are. Your happiness is yours to claim. Your power to keep yourself in a high-vibe state will help you be more successful, have deeper relationships, find balance and peace, feel fulfilled, prioritize your well-being, and always have the energy to give.

So where do we begin?

Awareness. Know what kind of state you're in. Words, both their presence and their absence, hold tremendous power (even in the form of thoughts). We can take them at face value, dig deep for meaning, or completely ignore them. What's important to remember is that they represent something— beliefs. Don't always believe the first things you tell yourself, especially if they're not constructive. It might be your old reflexes kicking in. We're here to evolve and train ourselves to have a feel-good reflex. The next chapters are going to teach you how to implement the five High Vibe Habits so you can let your best-self show up and guide you onwards and upwards.

If you do the same thing, day in and day out, you'll keep getting more of what you've got. If there's anything you'd like to have or feel more of (or less of), the High Vibe Habits will support you. Remember those negative, repetitive thoughts you have each day? Now you're going to transform them into a more constructive autopilot.

A big part of understanding ourselves and this practice is accepting fear instead of banishing it. You're going to retrain your mind to unlearn old meanings and turn down the volume on fear, so you can hear all your internal responses, not just one.

Courage is a currency. It's something I lend and something I borrow. I think a lot of what I have been able to do has been because I borrowed courage from others, like my family and friends, when I was running low. There's a cool part about this currency system; We never have to feel bad about borrowing because we always have enough to lend. It's like a secret stash that's not always available for us to have, but always available for us to give.

If this feels like a big undertaking, remember this: You're not alone. It's easy for me to believe in you. Borrow my courage. Courage has a curious way of attracting things, people, and opportunities (like this book!)—whatever it is you need.

66

When you talk, you are only repeating what you already know. But if you listen, you may learn something new.

—The Dalai Lama

THREE

CLARITY

You process up to seventy thousand thoughts a day[10]—eighty percent negative, ninety-five percent repetitive[11]. It's obvious, but I'm going to say it anyway—that's a lot of unproductive thoughts. And it doesn't end there. Those thoughts (and the actions they inform) that lead you astray aren't just unproductive, they're also *counter*productive. They're not just slowing you down, they're moving you away from what you actually want.

And that brings me to my first question: *What do you want?*

Clarity, as a habit, is the connection within so you can always answer that

---

[10] Healthy Brains by Cleveland Clinic. "*Brain Facts - Healthy Brains by Cleveland Clinic,*" May 11, 2020. https://healthybrains.org/brain-facts/.

[11] "*Stuck on Negative Thinking,*" n.d. Care Counseling. https://care-clinics.com/stuck-on-negative-thinking/.

question swiftly and surely. It's knowing that sometimes we must put something down (like those old beliefs), so we can pick something else up.

Whether you know what you want or just know you want something different, you're headed in the right direction. Not knowing is also information. It just requires more experimentation. Exploration leads to understanding your likes or dislikes. Either way the outcome keeps offering you guidance when you practice the process of clarity.

We are hours away from leaving for a family wedding and my daughter is desperate to have new shoes (the ones I'd promised her a while back). I'd put off the search hoping she would forget. She's in a growth spurt and the conscious consumer in me cringes at the idea of buying a pair of shoes she'll wear once.

But here we are at Nordstrom Rack with a dilemma on our hands. She's managed to find two pairs of shoes and feels strongly that she might "die" if she doesn't get them both. What's a mother to do?

This brings me to the first C of the High Vibe Habits. . . clarity.

What does shoe shopping have to do with this anyway? I'll tell you.

Clarity is something we tend to be more aware of when it comes to the big decisions in our lives: choosing a partner, buying a home, switching careers. But a lot of us are stuck in distracted living when it comes to the small ones.

We beat ourselves up over that extra slice of cake, binging Netflix on a weekday, or not making time to work out one day. None of these as stand-alone events changes anything. Except that our lives are mostly made up of these small events.

So why are we so hard on ourselves over these insignificant details? Because the small things are really small steps. Our choice to react or respond reflects our level of clarity. The small stuff doesn't need to be a big deal, but when we consistently stop showing up for what we want in the small things, we alter our trajectory.

When we are clear, we know our why, and making choices that move our goal needle is easy. We focus on what we gain rather than what we give up.

Meanwhile. . . back at Nordstrom Rack. . .

I weigh my options. I acknowledge my daughter's desire for both shoes. (I'm also a shoe person, so I really do understand her position.) I calmly tell her that she gets to choose one pair of shoes. And that one pair, while less than two, is still one more pair than she has now.

We go over the usual stuff, like our plan to buy only one pair, that we are working within a budget, and how we can practice shifting our focus and using gratefulness towards the one pair we are purchasing, instead of focusing on the one shiny pair we are leaving behind.

And then, I walked away.

I gave her time to process. Honestly, I needed the time to practice my breathing. I embarked on this errand thinking it would be quick, and this was beginning to feel frustrating to me. I was burning more time than I expected to. But my clarity on what I wanted for her outweighed my ego's need to use power.

There were tears and frustration, but in the end, she chose one pair and walked out with a smile. She learned she could make tough decisions. She learned to work within the constraints she had. She learned she could be grateful while wanting more. She left more confident in her abilities. And that, to me, was worth every minute we spent there.

I left feeling grateful for my clarity. I do not always make the aligned choice, but that day I did. And it felt so good. Parenting, like everything else in life, is one small action after another.

Making a small, aligned choice has a significantly larger emotional payout than you would expect. It shapes who we believe we are. It's another line we add to our story. What we believe about ourselves, and our abilities affects everything, big or small.

HIGH VIBE REFRAME

YOU ALWAYS HAVE A CHOICE - NOT IN WHAT HAPPENS TO YOU, BUT WHETHER YOU REACT OR RESPOND THOUGHTFULLY.

You are here.

Are you familiar with that dot or X on a map that helps you get your bearings? Well, consider this an official call to action to find your place—to identify where you are. Having clarity offers many empowering benefits. On top of knowing what you want, this habit actually gifts you the strength to reach that goal. Holding a clear vision means you find the tool, be it patience, motivation, or courage, to stay the course. Being able to stick with something is a huge contributing factor to success. Clarity and the other High Vibe Habits let us stay in the game *and* play our best game.

Learning how to recognize and then transform our current thoughts is to realize that our thoughts have a pattern, a sort of autopilot. We are more likely to have constructive thoughts when we are in a higher vibrational state (joy, love, peace, fun) and destructive thoughts when we're in a lower vibrational state (fear, stress, guilt, shame). Setting a course for a high-vibe life sets our default to a supportive and uplifting one. The trick is knowing how to stay there. The answer is the High Vibe Habits.

A quick reminder that the High Vibe Habits already lie within you. It might be that they've been dormant, maybe they're just a little dusty. You might be actively using them in one area of life but not in another. With this book, you're releasing the old habits you've been practicing that foster feelings of fear, lack, and stress. You're hitting pause by microdosing happiness so you can choose to nurture a higher vibrational state.

Those high-vibe states show you more possibility and open you up to low-stress perspectives.

HIGH VIBE REFRAME

YOU GET TO CHOOSE YOUR LIFE EXPERIENCE BY OFFERING YOURSELF WHAT YOU NEED.

Clarity is the first step we're going to take. Negative inner dialogue makes us less happy, healthy, productive, and effective. These thoughts waste two of your most precious resources: time and energy. I'm not going to tell you what to do, think, or feel. But I'll tell you that clarity will transform what you do, think, and feel to become so dialed into what you actually want that your very nature reflexively guides you there.

You get to want what you want. It doesn't mean it's convenient or easy or that anyone else will think it's a great idea. Clarity lets us redefine our goals and our values, so we can realign our thoughts and actions to create the life we want. Can we pause for a second? Because the idea of having a desire, a "want," isn't always welcome in our world. Throughout this chapter on clarity, we'll be talking about identifying what we want, but also the reframes we need to eliminate the blocks to make the High Vibe Habits our own.

HIGH VIBE REFRAME

DESIRES ARE
HIGH LEVEL NEEDS.

Meeting our desires isn't crucial for survival, but it is for thriving. Prioritizing our own needs, wants, and well-being requires us to value something that is of no value to anyone but us. That's how it feels anyway, which brings me to another point. . .

HIGH VIBE REFRAME

PRIORITIZING YOURSELF SUPPORTS YOUR ABILITY TO SUPPORT OTHERS.

It can be hard to get ourselves on board to consistently make space for ourselves in our lives.

It's even harder when we have to get other people on board to support our ability to do so. You get to show yourself an enormous amount of self-compassion as you go through this transformation. If you've been depriving yourself of health or happiness for a long time, it can feel impossible to account for the gap you perceive between where you are and where you'd like to be. But here's a comforting thought: It takes so much less than you think to get yourself to a better place. Consistency is key.

HIGH VIBE REFRAME

SMALL THINGS DONE WITH CONSISTENCY LEAD TO GIANT GAINS.

We can find clarity in our thoughts, actions, reactions, wants, and needs. Like Hansel and Gretel, we can follow the breadcrumb trail back to a belief that either blocks us or sets us free. (Beliefs are just thoughts we have over and over again until we take them for truths.) The more inquisitive and objective we are, the more we are open to seeing.

The two main buckets for this chapter are clarity of self and clarity of vision. Each time you work on these, you'll want to ask yourself these questions:

- How do I feel right now in this area?
- Where do I want to be or what do I want to feel? And where am I now?
- What might I be doing or thinking that's stopping me from having this?
- What would be good about having this or feeling this?

The questions expand our focal point to see beyond what's missing to include our desire and the steps to actualize it. It's the beginning of a simple shift in focus, from the empty spaces in our lives to the fullness that exists.

Clarity + Self

Self-clarity is so powerful because how we see ourselves changes how we show up in our lives. So many of the thoughts and decisions we make are based on perceived fears of losing what other people give us: love, connection, titles, prestige, admiration, security, community, and identity. We get stressed about what we do, say, and how we look and live because of what we believe someone else thinks. All this happens because we don't realize that we also get to offer ourselves these things. If we don't know what we are, it's up for discussion. When we feel uncertain or sensitive to the reactions and thoughts of others, it's almost always directly linked to the absence of offering ourselves that very thing.

I worked harder and harder in an unpleasant work environment to be seen as smart and successful. I've followed the rules so others would think I'm good. I've succumbed to conventional norms to feel pretty. I was driven to be what others wanted because I believed it was how I would feel whole, complete, and perfect. I eventually recognized a pattern. The comments and remarks that stung were the ones I didn't want to be true and the ones I feared might be true.

Simply put, self-clarity is knowing yourself on a deep level. At first glance, it may not appear to have any significant value. But it impacts every area of your life and all the choices you make. People will always tell us what we are and what we're not. But we don't have to believe it if we know the answer for ourselves. Having this "knowing" means we're diverting the time and energy from proving or defending ourselves to the decisions that move our goal needle.

So, what happens if during self-clarity you decide you're not exactly the person you want to be? Good news! It means you're human and have room to grow. That's it. You're not defective, deficient, or lacking; you're in training.

Exploring how we can objectively evaluate and define each of these traits is part of our unlearning. There have been people in my life who told me I wasn't generous. But I genuinely wanted to be a generous person. For years, all I would notice was stingy behavior. If I tipped someone, I would always feel guilty thinking I could've given more.

Any time money was involved I would feel poorly about myself, "knowing" that someone else would've done or given more than me.

But when I brought self-clarity into my life, I got curious and looked for all the ways I could be generous. I could give time, love, thoughts, and yes, money. When I let myself tally up my generosity in all these areas, I began to feel better. I also recognized that my discomfort with spending money wasn't about generosity but about my financial insecurity. Generosity is something I appreciate in myself and others. Knowing where I stood and accepting that I get to evolve brought me more confidence.

Self-clarity has two huge benefits. First, you get to be attuned to your feelings and emotions without suffering from them. Self-clarity allows you to sail through the world more smoothly. When something does catch you off guard, use it as an opportunity to know yourself better. Ask, *what am I questioning about myself?* Decide for yourself who you are, who you aren't, and who you want to be.

The second is you belong. You've got to spend time in the life you want before it can feel like home. When we reach, stretch, and grow, we leave our comfort zone and enter someplace new. The clarity of self-awareness lets us focus on being our best, versus wondering if we're good enough. The uncomfortable nature of expanding yourself isn't a sign you don't belong there—you're not an imposter. It's a sign you've entered a new arena. Sometimes we have people who support us and remind us that we've earned it or that we're enough. Their belief buoys us. And sometimes, other people believe your place is in the past, in the you from five years ago, the you from five minutes ago. And then, we must believe in ourselves. When we do that for ourselves, we help everyone else see it too.

Clarity + Vision

My husband is really supportive of my entrepreneurial life. He once told me to keep chasing my dreams and he'd be right behind me, supporting me. At first, I thought it was sweet.

But then the words lingered in my mind. . . *chasing a dream.*

Being a visual person, images came to mind. The first had me imagining I was running after a star, leaping, grasping, but always coming out empty-handed. The next was a game of tag. I ran and ran, trying different tactics of speed, patience, and strategy, but was never actually able to catch anyone. Both left me drained and with nothing in hand.

Language is power. That wasn't the experience I wanted to connect with my dreams. So, I thought, what about *growing* a dream?

When I grow something, I have a different approach. Cultivating is not at all the same as chasing. I let go of controlling the outcome and realized I could influence it instead. When I grow a garden, my effort is a really important contribution, but I don't have any guarantees about the outcome. Yet, I choose to do it anyway.

We pour ourselves into this venture. We show up. We might research. We learn how to support and grow this thing. There are so many factors that contribute to success. Soil quality, temperature, light exposure, pests. We don't automatically assume we're bad gardeners if we don't get it right the first time. Every outcome can make us better. Improvement comes from showing up and staying committed. This is true in any endeavor we undertake. Rather than feel defeated or exhausted, we experiment, seek advice, and try again. We happily stay in the game.

Vision-clarity is seeing an end goal and bringing it into focus. Zooming out lets you capture the essence of what you want in your life—the feelings. Living day to day makes it easy to forget that everything we are working for and towards offers us something: safety, security, fun, joy, legacy, or prestige. Once we understand what we want in our lives, we can zoom back in and identify how we're going to make it happen. Zooming in lets you figure out how to offer yourself a piece of that bigger feeling daily. If you're already doing this, great! There are ways you can keep evolving your practice for better results.

I encourage you to imagine yourself as a set of nesting dolls. Beginning as the smallest, you expand and grow to a larger and larger version of yourself. Our growth is infinite.

Through it all, the High Vibe Habits continue to serve us, always allowing us to expand and offering us something new at each iteration.

Steeping ourselves in our vision also signals to our brains to pay more attention to the things that matter. Sometimes we believe the things we crave don't exist in our lives. Clarity about what you want to bring into your life often gives you glimpses of how those things are already showing up. You're closer to the feelings in your vision than you expect. Witnessing even the smallest sliver of that desire can sometimes be enough to shift us from a feeling of desperation to exploration.

If you're looking for a romantic partner, you might begin to take note of all the love you get from your family and friends. If you're looking for a new job, you might become aware of how your current one is preparing you for something better. If you're looking for money, you might write down all the abundance that comes your way (love, time, discounts, gifts). You want things because of the feelings you expect them to bring. Love, security, freedom, community. So, find any bit of that future feeling that you're having right now and start to cultivate it. Take advantage of your confirmation bias. Your brain will start finding the things you value all around you.

Once you know what you'd like to nurture, you get to reverse engineer it into bite-sized portions. Big dreams are great, but they're kind of like a new roll of tape— finding where to start can be hard! But not starting is not an option. Breaking goals down, one step at a time, into tasks that can be completed in one sitting is what shows you that consistently taking small steps really will move mountains.

This falls under the vision umbrella because vision-clarity is your compass. The day-to-day can and probably will change as you experiment and adapt to stick with what works for you. You account for how the journey feels. And because of that, happiness isn't something you earn, it's how you live.

The Whole Effect

Armed with all this clarity, you've created a lighthouse for yourself. The journey is not a straight line, but your new guidepost identifies what you say yes to (your specific vision) and no to (no more shiny-object syndrome) and *not* feel bad about it. Having a deep understanding of your wants and needs is the first step to freedom from low-vibe emotions and the actions that follow. A lot of our energy is spent on activities that we take on because we thought we needed to say yes.

Clarity permits us to begin eliminating our drag. You trim away the things you do because you "should" do them, carving out the space for what needs to get done to live your best life. It makes a distinction between busy and productive. Being productive can keep you busy, but busy isn't always productive. Clarity allows decisions to be clear-cut—either they align with your goal or they don't. It's not about rigidity, but fluidity. Now, when you choose where to put your energy, you understand that it's moving you toward your goals (like strengthening a relationship, taking advantage of an opportunity, or saying no to a distracting "opportunity").

Look at saying 'no' as an efficiency skill. It's being able to understand what the cost of the ask is and hold that up against the goal. There are a lot of nuances to this skill, but with practice, you'll start to feel more comfortable. 'No' allows you to free up time because you can see how everything you do is an ask for resources. Before clarity, we default to sacrificing our wants and needs, always doing for others. After, we trust in the guidance of our compass. Following that path will bring us to what we desire to have, feel, and be. Guilt is a dirty opponent; the only way to win against it is to give in to it. Once we accept that our well-being is directly related to our ability to give to others, we can ask ourselves the important question: *How do I give in service instead of in servitude?* Clearly defining our role as we would like it to be—knowing our expectations—begins with asking ourselves, what does enough mean to me?

Feeling good is a direct win for you and an indirect win for everyone else. The investment you make in you flows through you to everyone else. Setting clear definitions and boundaries for yourself creates a distinct end result. When you can see the way, it feels more than possible. It feels probable. If slowing down or pausing to gain clarity feels impossible, that's probably the sign that now is exactly the time to do it. Clarity is an investment.

Here's another no-judgment reminder: Well-being is meeting both our wants and needs. Wants are high-level needs. If there's an ask coming from within you, it represents a need. Setting a thrive target means valuing things others may not and that's okay because it means something to you. This could apply to how you can value rest. I see it as an essential part of the productivity cycle. I make time to sleep and do everything I can (eat well, exercise, meditate) to set myself up for success in this area knowing my productivity benefits from it.

Knowing yourself deeply leads to so many desirable side effects. We become better decision-makers, less stressed, more efficient, empathic, happier, healthier, and inspired. We also become more effective communicators. Let's stick with this for a minute. Relationships contribute significantly to our happiness or our regret. Our interaction with the people around us determines which of these we're experiencing.

We are *always* communicating. And all communication has a purpose. You might be informing, teaching, connecting, advocating, supporting, loving, or even entertaining. I'm not suggesting you begin to dissect every word before it comes out of your mouth. Self-clarity and vision-clarity keep us tuned in to ourselves and how we relate to other people.

Most of us are in an autopilot setting, especially in familiar environments like our homes, workplaces, or with families. Autopilot saves energy, but it traps us in habitual behavior that doesn't always serve us. Do you find yourself feeling bad for the same behavior? Getting angry, not listening, or cutting people off mid-sentence can be habits. And even though we want the other person to feel heard, loved, and seen, we aren't communicating with that goal in mind.

Habits can also be hard to break because others expect us to show up in a certain way. When people know us as quiet, entertaining, passive, or decision-makers, there's the expectation that we'll always act according to those labels. But sometimes the quiet person wants to speak up. Sometimes the decision maker wants to just go along for the ride. This is why family gatherings can challenge us. We fall back into or are expected to, reenter the same dynamics as if time stood still. It can even happen under our roof after years of cohabitating.

A helpful way to switch things up is to change *your* perspective. In conversations, we so often attribute power to the speaker, but I encourage you to make listening less passive and more active. When we have self-clarity, I'm less affected by what other people are saying and doing. I'm more available to read between the lines and understand their motivation. And that changes my interpretation of the interaction. When it comes to communication, feeling seen and being heard are two essential parts of the human experience. They're things we long for and feel incomplete without.

Last year, I decided to switch up my son's piano teacher, which led to a frazzled email from the director of the program. I decided a quick call would be the least painful option, but my hairs stood on edge sensing the coming confrontation.

When I introduced myself, Dave immediately sounded defensive. He stuttered accusations at me, attempted to make me feel bad for my choice, and pointed out that I didn't read the contract. That last part was true—oops.

At first, I heard the defensive tone in my voice. I didn't want to be a pushover. I wasn't willing to feel guilty for the choices the school made. But then a High Vibe Habit kicked in. Something came over me: I got curious. As I listened to him, I began to ask myself, *how is Dave feeling? What is he really trying to tell me?*

I immediately detected hurt, frustration, and maybe even sadness. I apologized for the short notice, offered to continue for the three remaining weeks, and complimented the school and teacher. I laid out that this was a logistical issue for our family. From a genuine place in my heart, I asked him, "How can I make this feel good for you?"

And just like that, he melted. He understood, showered my son with compliments, and said he'd welcome us back with open arms should we choose to return.

Wow.

I couldn't believe the one-eighty he pulled, all because I heard him. I didn't have to inflate or deflate myself to make him feel better. He just needed to know that I understood him. This is how communication can be when we don't feel responsible for other people's feelings but instead feel compassion for them. Not adding my emotions let me powerfully see his. Communication often has a deeper meaning, though it may not always be clear. Improving our *intra*-communication skills improves our *inter*-communication skills.

I invite you to experiment with this in your personal or professional life. When your child gets upset, your spouse overreacts (or underreacts), or your coworker makes a comment, remember the power you hold. The way people respond and react is almost always about them, not you. Look for deeper meaning. Without diminishing your light, see theirs.

The people who suffer the most from our underdeveloped communication skills tend to be those we love the most. We can hear better and respond more accurately when there's less noise in our minds. And clarity does that. It lets the swirling thoughts settle, creating space to actively listen. Taking the time to get clear on how I want to show up and what I want the other person to feel transforms relationships. It breaks the cycle of treating loved ones poorly or unfairly. It makes us more open to receiving feedback and growing. When we hear what other people need, we know how to show up for them.

Sometimes my husband and I feel like ships passing in the night. Our brief time overlap becomes precious. When my mind buzzes with to-do lists and worries, I don't listen well. I don't mean to, but I tune out. Clarity brings my values and old habits to the surface. I choose to become more intentional with my interactions. I stop. I make eye contact. I ask questions. I reflect on what I hear. All this engagement helps me communicate my love by offering my whole self. The same goes for my children, colleagues, friends, and strangers. Being a good communicator (which happens when we speak *and* when we listen) is a role where we both give and receive.

None of this is to make excuses for our own or other people's behavior. I'm not suggesting you tolerate or bend to other people's mistreatment. And I don't think apologizing for our behavior only to do it on repeat is what any of us want. Keep your boundaries but learn how to glean clarity.

Progress over perfection dissolves any fear lingering inside that we might regret what became of our relationships. Show up in the small, everyday moments.

Exploring Blocks

How matters. So, as you start setting a high-vibe intention, view the process as an exploration. To effectively create a new constructive habit, you need to know what it's replacing so you can identify when you're practicing an old habit. We just covered the benefits of clarity and how to start cultivating them. But what gets in the way of clarity? Changing our thoughts has us pushing up against some of the norms of our society. Prioritizing our well-being means investing resources in things that have no direct benefit to others. We're basically asking ourselves to be comfortable doing what most of society defines as selfish. No big deal, right? Our reflexes might still inject this idea into our minds: If I'm not giving, I must be taking. Here's the advice I give myself, especially on the hard days. *Don't believe everything you tell yourself.* Certainly not when it comes to that first negative thought.

Replacing habits means we should get good at recognizing our blocks as the unproductive habits that they are.

Let's explore some of the common blocks you might be turning to. Seeing your block clearly is how you know what you can stop doing. If you feel some pushback on your new path, know you're probably on the right path, not the wrong one.

Compare and Despair

First up, comparison culture. We are all at different stages and places in our lives, but comparison tells us to pick the ideal and hold ourselves to that standard. And to do so almost illogically, like comparing apples to oranges. Comparison gives us a chance to feel better or worse than someone else. It's one way to find value in our lives, but it means living relative to everyone else. Last time I checked, it's pretty easy to look around and find ourselves in someone else's shadow, eclipsed by their achievements or character. High-vibrational states let us focus on progress, or competition with ourselves, as a way of identifying value in our lives. The real cost of comparing ourselves is self-acceptance and enjoying our choices.

For every choice we make, someone else is making a very different choice *and* making it look good. Comparison is like selective hearing. We are choosing to take a snippet of someone's life and use it to create a whole story from which we compare our own lives. This isn't something we just do on social media. We do this more than we realize. I've gone on a beach vacation and been lulled into the beauty and pace of that lifestyle. I've gone to parties and met extremely accomplished individuals living fascinating lives. A part of me is attracted to a part of each of those lifestyles. But if I compare my life to theirs as a whole, I could feel like my life is never good enough. It's not chill enough at one end and not ambitious enough at the other. The sliver I witness while on vacation or the story I romanticize at a cocktail party is not an accurate representation of the life choices I would have to make to have those lifestyles. We forget that each comes with a unique path. Every outcome is built from a lifetime's worth of choices that it takes to get there. Instead, we can choose to be inspired to find our version of what we see. I could find time to slow down, and I could find a way to feed my thirst for a more accomplished life. There's no right or wrong choice, just what's right for you. We rob ourselves of the joy of our choices if we are looking for joy from someone else's. It's a never-ending story of lack because there will always be someone making a different choice and living a different life.

When I first chose to stay at home with my children, I had people lovingly ask me why I was wasting my talents. Ouch. I had known for a long time that staying at home was something I deeply wanted. Because I wasn't sure how to feel good about choices that others didn't approve of, I felt hurt by these comments. I felt confused. I felt less valuable. I felt compelled to prove to everyone that I could stay at home and not squander my talents. Who was I to waste the privilege I was blessed with?

Soon after my second child, an opportunity presented itself and I accepted. It was a wonderful founding role, and I wasn't going to let a little thing like timing get in the way. But a good thing at the wrong time is rarely great. I knew the experience I was having was falling short of the mothering experience I wanted and wanted to offer my children. And I was always afraid I was falling short as a cofounder. I could never do enough or be enough to either. Being physically present with my children wasn't enough to always be mentally present or to have the breathing room to do more than the life-sustaining and managerial tasks involved with raising two small children. I had partial clarity. I knew I wasn't going to give up being at home with my children. But I couldn't accept I was in a stage with high emotional and physical demands. Another example of the dangers of partially believing in ourselves has us out on a limb without our flight feathers. A stage by definition is a passing time. Children grow and, while they might always need their parents, ask different things from us. Acceptance would have allowed me to feel comfortable acknowledging there was time for both family and work, but just not yet.

Notice the stage you're in and find the positive within it, rather than always wishing to be somewhere else. Or someone else. Internal conflict often robs us of the joy around us at any given moment. Taking a day off is hardly enjoyable or valuable if you spend the day thinking of how you should be doing something more productive.

Remember my son's ice cream sandwich? We are more likely to enjoy the choices we make when we are clear on what we want and believe in the value of our decisions. This block pertains to clarity because chasing doesn't feel like progress. I can't reach a goal if I keep changing the target.

Expectation and Guilt

The second block is around expectation that leads to guilt. That's the "should" feeling we often operate from instead of the want. How you feel changes what giving feels like. It can make things easy or make us exhausted and bitter. Have you ever done a favor for someone when your tank felt empty? Maybe you're spending time with someone, and you find yourself spacing out or doing things grumbling under your breath. You might feel overextended and overwhelmed thinking about what's left on your long to-do list. You've probably also been on the receiving end and felt that difference. Have you ever needed someone's help and felt guilty because they're clearly not happy about helping? Putting ourselves in the recipient's shoes lets us get more clarity on why we want to show up more intentionally. Again, this judgment-free zone we create lets us explore our habits by getting curious about all our experiences. Everyone wins when we know how to give from a high-vibe state.

Being driven by other people's expectations of us overshadows our ability to hear our voices and meet our own needs. Guilt, shame, and regret are really powerful oppressors. The fear they create within us leaves us scrambling to meet our needs and makes personal desires feel selfish. Living by 'should' can make us resentful and lead us to burnout and declining physical health. In her book *Wolfpack*, Abby Wambach beautifully illustrates how we can understand ourselves as individuals within our family and community. She says, "The strength of the pack is the wolf, and the strength of the wolf is the pack." We are all connected. Caring for your well-being contributes to your capacity to support others.

Humans survive because of community, but we thrive with the *right* community. This doesn't mean that you stop doing things for others. It means you don't stop doing things for yourself. You learn that giving is a two-way street: from you and to you. That's how you give from a place of overflow rather than depletion. High-vibe states create a regenerative energy source within you, leaving you with more to offer everyone around you.

This block affects your clarity because you can't hear what you want if all you hear is what other people want.

Stuckness

Why is it so hard to change course? Doing more of the same is easy, comfortable, and predictable. But there's also the sunk-cost fallacy. This is the idea that we choose not to change course or direction, even if it benefits us because we've already committed to it. It might look like finishing a book that you aren't enjoying. It might be as big as staying in a career you don't love because you've already spent years in it or invested in an education for it. Sometimes we're aware that we've fallen prey to this fallacy, but sometimes we aren't.

Distracted living habits tend to make us feel stuck by distorting and diminishing the value of change. Maybe it's due to our brains' desire to conserve energy, maybe it's because we feel safe with what we know. There's a satisfaction we feel when we complete something. I've seen it in children, and I've experienced it as an adult. But life isn't something to complete or check off. It's something to experience. When we begin to apply that "completion-equals-satisfaction" thought process across the board, we can fall prey to the sunk-cost fallacy. We act stuck because we feel stuck.

Culture, society, and family can all reinforce our steadfastness. Convincing yourself to change can be hard. Convincing everyone around you can make change feel impossible. There are lots of payoffs to stay the course. It's hard, "wasteful," and scary, especially if it means doing something less conventional or following a calling. It's hard to give ourselves the permission to change our minds. In the beginning, it can look more like confusion than clarity.

When I applied to law school, I had a lot of momentum behind that choice. I studied hard, took the LSAT, filled out applications, and worked as a paralegal. I tried to ignore the fact that I might actually want something different. Forces invisible to me made me feel rooted. I knew it was an approved path. The constrictive nature of distracted living made me feel committed and made it difficult for me to feel open to accepting what I knew felt right—*not* going to law school. Thankfully, I had support and encouragement (thanks, Mom!) which gave me the courage to contemplate another option. Fear of change is so often a fear of the unknown and maybe even a fear of failure.

We don't lose our desire simply because we don't act on it. Left abandoned, it gnaws at us. We notice its absence as we look at others' lives and back to our own. Choosing to follow your clarity might feel scary, but ignoring it has its risks. Feeling poorly often feels more normal and more acceptable than the alternative, but it doesn't have to be your story.

You get to want what you want. And you get to change your mind (and your course) when you feel like it's not working. Every situation is unique, but sometimes it's more important to be committed to the vision than the current plan. This block denies us clarity because if we are more invested in the path than the destination, we end up exactly where we planned, but not exactly where we wanted. If we continue down a path without knowing if it's our path to health and happiness, we risk living a life that doesn't offer us what we need.

Sourcing Information

We're all pretty used to receiving and looking for information outside of us. But clarity is a habit of tuning into your *intra*communication skills. And that means tuning into what comes *from* you, not just to you. Intuition, desire, and gut feelings don't always feel like legitimate sources of information if we aren't used to trusting them. Our body and mind are always sending us signals helping us identify how we feel and what we want. These are powerful clarity tools.

As I mentioned earlier, all feelings provide us with information. These things come with the physiological sensations that offer our brain information. Information we might want to bring into our decision-making process. It's valuable to utilize all the incoming messages we receive from ourselves. Even if your mind isn't articulating your needs, your body is likely sending you physical signals. If you've ever experienced knots or butterflies in your stomach, your throat tightening, or sweating, translate the sensations and take them into account. I'm not saying that you need to make all your decisions based on them, but you'll want to allow them to weigh in.

The distracted habits of learned deprivation teach us to repeatedly tune into specific emotions like fear, amplifying their voices and drowning out the others that could balance them out. The High Vibe Habits aren't for eliminating any emotions. They teach us to identify this overstimulation, seek out the other things we feel, and hear the other thoughts we have.

I believe that well-being is achieved when we are meeting our needs and our wants. When we don't spend enough time in the clarity phase and dig deep enough, it's easy to ignore our desires because we don't recognize them. We're constantly being bombarded with other people's opinions making it difficult to trust our own voice. We confuse the beliefs that we adopted to be the ones we decided for ourselves. That's how we sometimes end up unfulfilled, even after we've attained that "thing," be it a job, family, house, car, salary, or goal.

This block affects our clarity because we need access to all the information possible to have full clarity and to remember that each of us is being guided by an internal intelligence.

Let's recap. Clarity gets your minds working for you. It lets you get in the driver's seat with your confirmation bias. It helps you connect to your desire and often find that a piece of what you're looking for is already in your life. It also shows you that you might be creating the blocks to your happiness. Identifying all these blocks is what helps you stay high vibe.

Uncovering Clarity

How do we glean clarity? Clarity is everywhere. We have to pause to see it, which is why microdosing happiness is our stepping stone. It can come from what we don't want or from what we do want, from negative or positive experiences.

One of those moments from my early twenties was an evening that is still fuzzy in detail but crystal clear in its lesson.

I felt impatient as I waited under an ugly orange glow. It probably made me look as bad as I felt. I was overstimulated from all the music, alcohol, and conversation. I didn't even want to know what time it was. All I knew was that I could already feel the exhaustion, dehydration, and gastritis punishing me for yet another routine night out in New York City. My feet hurt and I was dying to just get into a cab and go home. My boyfriend (now husband) continued talking to his friend on the corner as I waited. . .

That's the last detail that we can both agree on. I don't know if it's fair for me to tell you the rest of my version of it. Like all events that occur when both parties are inebriated, what I can recount is my foggy version. It's a night we brought up a few times afterward, but it never lost its sting for either of us, so we agreed to disagree and put it behind us.

Here's what I know for sure though. Neither of us showed up as our best selves. In fact, I'd say that evening brought out the ugly in both of us (and it wasn't because of the nasty street lamp lighting).

That night somehow represented everything I'd been working *not* to bring into my life: anger, pettiness, exhaustion, distrust. Something needed to change. I had to let go of the idea of being controlling. I couldn't change my partner's behavior, choices, or memory. It's one of the first times I can remember understanding that regaining control of my life meant I needed to change. We could've kept fighting. That would've been the easy thing to do. But as impossible as letting go felt, I had the clarity to choose the future I wanted.

This is an example of how showing up as less was altering my trajectory. Self-clarity would've filled me with different feelings that led to different choices and different outcomes. Maybe I wouldn't have even been out that night. And that brings me to another orange streetlamp on a completely different night. This time, a positive clarity moment unfolded—my twenty-third birthday.

What a night to be in the West Village. It was a cold, but beautifully crisp December evening. My mother and I were chatting, fluffy snowflakes gently falling onto my eyelashes. We were in line for an amazing sushi spot in New York City. I peeked around the couple in front of us. We were still several people away from reaching the clear plastic extension all the restaurants add on during the winter months. The bright lights and bustling sounds of the city surrounded us, but we were so excited to be together that it all faded into the background. We chatted as easily about the latest fashion trends as we did about life's purpose.

As we shifted from foot to foot to keep warm, she asked me, "If it didn't matter how much you made or how risky it felt, what would you do?"

"I'd be a fashion designer!" It jumped out faster than I'd expected. I'd been a paralegal for the last year, prepping for law school. Lately, I'd had the unsettling feeling that this wasn't the path my heart would choose. But I liked making a plan and sticking to it. Besides, design school seemed uncertain and the industry highly competitive. Would I even be able to get a job?

"Then do it!" My mother beamed.

It feels surreal to say it, but I took her advice, attended Parsons School of Design, and got hired as a designer before I graduated. I felt such deep clarity during that conversation. I borrowed courage from my mother to take action (that's our next C, control). There were so many challenges along the way, but the confidence I felt from following my heart and doing the work grew daily. Because it felt right— *felt good*—I had more to put behind the desire.

There are positive ripples that come from aligned decisions. I was in the right place—a design job that I adored (unlike my *The Devil Wears Prada* experience). I woke up excited every single day and that energy made me stand out at work. I felt challenged positively. I learned to push myself to be more visible and believe in myself. Everything about my work was expanding me.

Looking back, I can see the beginnings of my constructive elements at work. This was a dream job. I felt like I had it all; I had work that I loved, a supportive community, and encouraging mentors. But without a consistent practice, these positive ripples didn't last. Without the protective support of my 5 C's, distractive elements (like imposter syndrome) crept in and began to rob me of joy, limiting my career potential. Distractive elements like comparison and judgment became obstacles keeping me from putting myself out there. Comparison and lack detracted from my ability to connect with my peers, who began feeling like my competition.

Having feelings of success only to have them melt away and reveal our insecurities can make us feel like there's something wrong with us. It provides our negative beliefs with the confirmation that we aren't good enough. It starts a negative cycle that usually ends in a self-fulfilling prophecy. A lot of us experience life as a rollercoaster ride of feeling good and then feeling lousy. So many of us, in fact, that we think it's normal and unavoidable. I know that ride. This work, my High Vibe Habits, was something I needed. But now they're something I get to share. No one should have to ride a rollercoaster of emotions and worthiness.

If you've been reading along this whole time and thinking this is great for other people, "But what about me? I don't even know what I want." I've got you. And you've already got some clarity just being able to know this about yourself. We're all starting in a different place, so if you're using other people as your metric, that's the old habit of comparison creeping in and making you feel low. Take a deep breath.

The first step is to realize that you might be experiencing a block or void. It might happen because you've never explored this idea before. Our desires can be buried, or they might not feel allowed or possible. Maybe what you seek is off-limits within the community you live in. If you don't feel like you're allowed to want what you want, it might be hiding from you on purpose. If it's an idea that feels like it would cause a lot of upheaval in your life (like changing careers or partners), we can be unwilling to see it. None of us wants the road to feeling good to be paved with a series of painful or difficult acts.

Wherever you are, just start by noticing where you feel good or not-so-great in your life. With curiosity, just spend a week or two taking notes on things that feel good and things that don't. Small is the perfect place to start. Just starting with one of those observations is how you know when to begin to microdose happiness. You've noticed how you're feeling. Now you get to ask yourself, "what can I do to feel better?" (That small thing you do to feel better is the art of microdosing happiness.) Remember, if you don't know what you want, you get to practice choosing something and testing out how that feels. The goal is to shift from focusing on *I don't know what I want* to experimenting and following the tiniest yeses you hear. Maybe it's a voice saying I'd like to sit in the sun for five more minutes. Maybe it's realizing you feel a little longing when you sign your child up for pottery class. Maybe it's how you pause on an Instagram post of dreamy destinations. The answers aren't hard to find if you're willing to ask yourself the questions and listen to what comes from inside of you.

Each day is an opportunity to live and contributes to the life you build. How you see yourself matters.

There's a parable about three bricklayers all working side by side. The architect stops to ask the first one, "What are you doing?"

He answers, "I'm a bricklayer. I'm working hard laying bricks to feed my family."

The second bricklayer is asked the same question. He answers, "I'm a builder. I'm building a wall."

The third, when posed with the same question, exclaims, "I'm a cathedral builder. I'm building a great cathedral to the Almighty."

What's your role and what are you building?

Our choices create value of some kind. Clarity lets us understand if it's actually where we want to be investing. Rather than be afraid that we can't do it all, approach life by doing what matters most. We inevitably give up one thing when we choose another. If I travel a lot, I may be less connected to my community. If I work a lot, I may have less time for my family. If I'm spending time with family, I may have less time to advance my career. There's an opportunity cost for everything in life. A 'yes' vote always casts a 'no' for something else. I'm not here to tell you what you can or can't do, be, or have. I'm here to help you realize that maybe there's something you haven't seen yet within you or around you.

Knowing what you want is how you can avoid the negative pull towards guilt, comparison, judgment, and ultimately, regret. Does working provide your family with the lifestyle you want to offer them? Does staying at home? It's not about what you choose in the end. It's about how you view that decision. And what you do with it. Practicing a habit of clarity intentionally sets your focus on what you are bringing to the table.

There was a time when Google Photos could trigger a sense of despair in me. Those "one year ago today" collages made me tear up and feel like I was doing something wrong. How could I be working from home and staying at home with my kids and still feel like I was missing the experience of being with them?

HIGH VIBE REFRAME

CLARITY IS HOW YOU STOP SEEING YOUR LIFE AS COSTS AND START SEEING IT IN TERMS OF INVESTMENTS.

I realized that sometimes my high ideals cost me the things I valued because of my desire to check boxes. I wanted my children to eat healthy homemade meals, but I also wanted them to have a calm and present mother. Food has always been one of my passions. Cooking is a creative outlet and way I express my love. But when I was sleep-deprived and spread thin, my insistence on made from scratch also made me more stressed and less present. I was physically there without always being mentally there. I was the busy bricklayer focusing on the wall, forgetting I was really here to build a cathedral. And it was exhausting because I was doing the work without receiving the real benefit. The price you pay for avoiding clarity work is regret. We can't get back what's behind us, but we can determine what lies ahead.

Time always gets filled because you must spend it. Your choice is to decide what you'll do with it. We can worry less about how to manage time if we learn to manage ourselves. We do that best when we have clarity.

HIGH VIBE REFRAME

WHEN WE MANAGE OUR MINDS, WE
MANAGE OUR TIME.

It's easy to believe that more time is the sole answer. But time's limited supply is actually what pushes us to find meaning and purpose, build relationships, and step out of our comfort zones. It's precisely because we don't know how much time we have, that (with clarity) we understand our priorities. More time isn't the whole answer, but the idea of more might be. Not squeezing more *in* but learning to squeeze more *out*. Feeling tired, exhausted, overworked, or underwhelmed with life are all low-vibe states that have us seeing ourselves and the world through different lenses.

Internal conflict creates confusion. When we get too exhausted from being cut down (and cutting ourselves down), we don't have the energy or motivation to change direction. Indecision can grip us because no 'right' or 'good' solution presents itself. The one we choose is usually the one where we sacrifice our own needs because, while it doesn't feel good, it does feel easier. And sometimes easy creates the short-term win we need. We all want to make decisions with ease and feel good about them. In the long term, those feel-good decisions are aided by clarity from knowing both what we've done and what we want.

Clarity and all the C's are habits we layer, mix, and reuse. They are always relevant because after we cycle through them, we find ourselves someplace new. As you evolve, what they unlock for you changes. These are tools, not a patch job. My clients are always excited when they share with me how the C's keep being useful. As you practice them, you are retraining your thought process little by little and you find yourself living more constructively. You transform your life each time you generate a new thought or redirect an unhelpful one. The success of my framework lies in its simplicity, which allows for consistency.

Creating The Habit

If we aren't moving towards what we want, we are moving away from it. Without clarity, our efforts and energy are often counterproductive. We've covered areas you can find clarity in, blocks your old habits might be creating, and strategies to sustain your high-vibe state.

How you feel changes your life because it changes what you do. Making a small, aligned choice has a significantly larger emotional payout than you would expect. It shapes who we believe we are. It's another line we add to our story. What we believe about ourselves, and our abilities affects everything, big or small. We make those right-for-us choices with clarity. Small and consistent steps create momentum. It gives us a healthy way to not only measure our progress but witness it. And that lets us feel good, which gives us motivation and all the other mental resources to keep going.

Clarity helps you feel grateful for what you have and what you've created so far. Now it's time to task it with the job of helping you thrive. That's an area you might have your sights set on—happiness, health, wealth, peace, and fulfillment—but not your habits. Clarity helps you keep finding and transforming your old beliefs, a.k.a. blocks, that stop you from actualizing your dreams. It creates alignment. A high-vibe life has desirable side effects. You don't just get happy, healthy, productive, and efficient. You stay that way. It's life amplified. The High Vibe Habits keep you feeling good, avoiding those chronic stress and fear zones, and giving you access to your most powerful level of brain activity to support yourself and the people in your life.

Stop waiting for another time, opportunity, or person to be the answer. Create the life you want today. It starts with you. Just like you'd review your academic or business performance quarterly or annually, see this clarity time as the investment that it is. Check in and stay tuned in to the vision you have for yourself and your life. Thinking consumes more energy than doing. Clarity practices (self-clarity and vision-clarity) give you more momentum as you roll into the action phase. Gifting yourself clarity means connecting to your why. And that leads to taking the right-for-you action you seek (which is the next C: control).

Here's the breakdown for clarity:

CLARITY encourages:
happiness, health, acceptance, perspective, vision, responsiveness, self-compassion, excellence, solution–oriented mindset, generosity, achievement, purpose, courage, inspiration, motivation, empathy, connection, peace

---

CLARITY **eliminates**:
perfectionism, overwhelm, indecision, reactiveness,
internal conflict, exhaustion, hustle culture, fear-
based overthinking, external pressure, jealousy,
regret, comparison, guilt, judgment

Avoid ever feeling lost, confused, or overwhelmed by beginning with the first C— clarity. Exercising your clarity habit starts with *asking*:

1. What am I doing now?

2. What do I want?

(If you don't know what you want, identify what you would like less of and then pick something you could try out for question two.)

And have you *believing*:

1. I serve others better when I serve myself.
2. Clarity shows me the small consistent steps I can take to make the progress I desire.

EXERCISES + INSIGHTS

This is a great time to start releasing that old habit of judging where you are and what you do. Learning how to observe yourself with a little detachment is a much more powerful skill.

These exercises are transformative because they help you rewire for a more constructive thought process. These habits are all about feeling good, so make practicing them as fun as possible. You can undertake a high-vibe transformation as a solo mission. But, community, even if it's just one other person, can contribute to momentum. It helps make us more accountable to ourselves. If it feels good, invite a friend along for a shared high-vibe journey.

Self-Clarity

Understanding who we are changes what we think is possible in our lives. We are often fueled by these invisible forces driving us to prove our worth, look for acceptance and acknowledgment from others, and avoid our fear of not being enough. Taking some time to decide who we are and how we want to show up makes decision-making surprisingly easy. It releases you from guilt by understanding that you are an energy conduit. When you care for yourself, you pass those benefits along to others. You can now see your needs as a priority because your well-being is an integral part of how you show up in every part of your life.

Giving In Service

Giving from a depleted place is very different than giving from a full cup. Giving can be a source of fulfillment in life, but not when obligation and 'should' are the dominant motivation. This is an excellent way to begin to separate yourself from that habit of guilt.

- What are others expecting of me?

- What's my expectation of myself?

- Am I trying to live into someone else's idea of what I should be doing?

- Do I have unrealistic expectations of myself?

NOTES

Should Versus Want

Make two columns in your journal titled "should" and "want" and start organizing your thoughts and activities accordingly. Remember that some things might feel like "should" initially but might be "want." For example: caring for an elderly parent. This can be a heavy responsibility, but it may also be something you want to do for your parent. Same for caring for your children. A "want" doesn't mean it's easy, but it is something that aligns with your values.

An example of a "should": keeping my house spotless because my friend manages to. My "want" may be clean versus spotless. I can be okay with a different standard because it lets me have more time or lets my family be more relaxed. Joy might be my bigger "want".

Now's your chance to assess your desire and motivation. Ask:

- What are you doing that is actually moving you closer to what you want?

- What are you doing that maintains an image, yours or someone else's?

NOTES

Journaling

You have about seventy-thousand thoughts per day, with eighty percent of them being negative, and ninety-five percent of them being repetitive. This week, gather information through awareness. Close your eyes, take a deep breath, and really hear your thoughts. Write them down. Seeing your thoughts on paper allows you to have a different relationship with them. You might find that some are outdated. Seeing similar thoughts repeatedly alerts you to a specific area you want to start to understand more. Ask:

- What do I have?

Gratefulness is a wonderful practice to experience the joy of what's already in our life. It's not a stopping point; it's a starting point. A lot of times we can find a piece of what we're working towards in our life, and awareness of that gift helps us stay inspired and motivated.

- What have I already created in my life that makes me feel good?

- What are the relationships in my life that   bring me joy?

- What am I already doing for my well-being (like reading this book!)?

NOTES

With a plan in hand, you're ready to take action. And that's exactly what we're going to talk about in the next chapter!

For more Clarity exercises, visit www.nithyakaria.com/highvibebook.

66

The task is not to control the wind, but to direct the movements of the ship so that it stays on course.

—Unknown

FOUR

CONTROL

"1-2-3. . . 1-2-3. . ."

"Come here!" she excitedly motions to me. I take up the space in front of my mother and find her arms resting on my shoulder and hip.

"1-2-3. . . 1-2-3. . ." We go gliding across the speckled wheat tiles in our foyer. I let her lead me round and round. I giggle as my steps try to follow her lead. She's always excited to teach me her latest ballroom dancing lesson. From the waltz to the foxtrot, none of the dance steps she taught me were a straight line. The beauty was in the fancy footwork that led us this way and that way. And I was always surprised how much ground we could cover in what initially felt like just going in a tiny circle.

Life is a lot like my impromptu dance lessons. We don't get anywhere only using the gas pedal. We rarely drive, or dance, only in a straight line. The beautiful journey we take has twists and turns, stop and go, highs and lows. Most of us get to our destination via the scenic route. But I'm thinking back to those dance steps. Every step we took sideways, forward, or backward was with purpose. The change in direction was never a loss of control. Control isn't about everything going the way you expect. It's about you being aware of your choices at all times.

HIGH VIBE REFRAME

THE DIFFICULTY WITH CONTROL ISN'T GETTING IT, IT'S KNOWING YOU ALREADY HAVE IT.

Even if we can't control the song that's playing, we can go back and forth in our ways with control to get to where we want to be. Simple isn't always easy. My mission is for this chapter to make it easier until it is easy. Because that's the thing about a habit, good or bad: once it's yours, it comes with ease.

No Way Out

There's simply no way out of making a decision, so the best thing is to set yourself up to make good decisions easily. Even when you're too tired to make another decision, you're making a decision. Even if you let someone else make the decisions, you're choosing to follow along. But that means that even when you aren't choosing something intentionally, *you are still choosing*. Just because you aren't aware of it doesn't mean you aren't exercising it. Every time you make a choice; you have the chance to recognize you have control in your life.

Even those unhelpful thoughts that pop into your head, over time, can change. And as you're building those new mental pathways, you always have a choice of what to listen to, what to change, and what to act on. How many times have you used the excuse that you just "are" something? I've heard *I'm just a yeller. I could never be that patient. I'm just a negative person*. And while we believe we are set in our ways; we spend a lot of energy hoping someone else will change. Control can feel like backward logic. It's something we don't believe is possible to have over ourselves, but something we feel is possible to exert over others.

Permission + Perspective

Control is about what we do (which is giving), but it's equally about receiving. Choosing what beliefs you continue to hold on to, and permitting yourself to hold more supportive and fair ones, lets you create balance in your life. It's the permission to invest in your health and happiness and create space for yourself in your own life, for your wants and needs.

There's no shortage of information about how to take care of yourself. But there's not a lot of support around carving out the time for it all. We can learn the time-saving strategies, but do you have the underlying support you need to make a radical shift in your thinking to: *I matter*? Believing "I matter" is the missing piece to living a life that feels good. It's how we consistently show up for ourselves and do the small things, day in and day out, amidst the constant requests for our time, energy, and finances. It's how we uphold the boundary that protects us from burnout, resentment, exhaustion, and emptiness.

Happy On Purpose

You get to decide what kind of life experience you have. It's a surrender of everything but your thoughts, beliefs, words, and actions. If you don't already practice this perspective habitually, it's difficult to believe it's enough. It opens the door to a world where you aren't underneath it all, bearing the weight on your shoulders. It's the high vantage point, the chance to live life with a top-down perspective instead of a bottom-up one. We are more aware, grateful, and generous from this place.

Control is the second of the High Vibe Habits. The habit is to shift your energy from trying to control things outside yourself to being in control of just yourself. Letting go, believe it or not, helps us feel more in control. This internal shift allows you to be a force that manifests desired changes around you, beginning from a powerful space within you.

Sometimes it's easier to understand something by knowing what it isn't. We can feel out of control when we don't achieve a certain outcome, that "should." A lot of what we spend our energy feeling bad about, within us or outside of us, revolves around measuring things against a preset standard. Good (or right) on one side and bad (or wrong) on the other. We can judge ourselves for anything and everything. I'm supposed to look like this, my kids are supposed to act like this, my partner is supposed to think like this—and it never ends. We never stop having this expectation of what life is supposed to look like. At an early age, we paint a "should" picture. It's the life other people want for us, expect from us, and teach us to strive for. Planning and expectation can easily have us believing we can predict the future and then feeling a loss of control when things go differently.

But I'm here to help you get clear on what the true domain of control is—yourself. And its purpose—to help you create and live the life you want. That includes feeling in control of your beliefs, thoughts, and actions. Everything else is *influenced* by these things.

You always have a choice, not in what happens to you, but in what you do with what happens. You get to decide how you think, feel, and respond. You create the meaning in your life and the reality you live. You choose your perspective. Each of the High Vibe Habits is simple and effective because it offers you a new, healthy way to see things. When you have that lens, you begin a chain reaction of automatic responses that support you in living the life you want. It's like a domino effect, where the High Vibe Habits are the first domino you tip in a positive sequence of choices, thoughts, and actions.

I have no doubt that you have accomplished a great many things in your life. Relish those wins. I'm not here to judge how you live your life. I'm offering you another perspective. Your life can feel and be the way you want even if it doesn't look exactly the way you imagined it would. In practicing control, you surrender the "my way is the only way," but you allow something else in. By redirecting your energy toward your own beliefs, thoughts, and actions, you allow yourself to feel a new sense of empowerment. It brings in a sense of security, safety, and predictability, knowing that you can create stability in your own life regardless of what comes your way. You build an internal trust bridge.

HIGH VIBE REFRAME

REALIZING YOUR CIRCLE OF CONTROL IS YOURSELF INCREASES YOUR SENSE OF STABILITY IN THE WORLD.

Spending energy on external factors tends to make us feel like we're playing defense. Juggling is the metaphor that comes to mind. You can't stop and sustain the act. It hinges on your constant effort. Progress feels difficult because you're stuck. We play a stronger offense through self-control, deciding what we'll do and how we'll feel regardless of anyone else.

Learning what to let go of and what to grab onto is the dance of control. Tightness, rigidity, being closed off, and absolute authority are by-products of being controll*ing*. Being in control has more to do with trust, knowing, and peace.

The good news is you can stop wanting to be in control. You're in the driver's seat, my friend! This chapter is going to show you how to build your habit of control and get intentional.

In the previous chapter, you spent time clarifying your direction, wants, and needs. Welcome to the execution phase, sandwiched between the planning and reflection phases, this is where your plan comes to life. You've prepped and plotted your new course, and now you need to get moving with aligned action. Aligned action is when what you do moves you closer to what you want. It's energy well spent on progress.

This step allows you to build a trust bridge with yourself. When you invest in clarity and then take the laid-out action steps, you're proving to yourself that you are capable of creating what you want in your life. It's very powerful to experience supporting yourself; you're giving yourself a chance to see that all the scary what-ifs your mind can come up with aren't so scary. Sometimes bad stuff happens, but so much of what blocks us is perceived fear. Scaring ourselves into the safety of avoiding change is a reflex supported by our negativity bias, which is happy to remind us of every time we've messed up. But scaring ourselves into stuckness doesn't make it feel any better.

Most of us just wake up one day and instead of choosing our day, it chooses us (classic distracted living). This happens as we add more and more elements into our lives: careers, romantic partners, children, and aging parents. They bring us joy, but then they begin to run our lives. Our desires (connection to family, marriage, careers, starting our own family) devolve into the list of acts that come with the roles. That list snowballs into something that often feels bigger than us. Forget being able to enjoy all the pieces of our lives, we end up spending our energy trying not to get steamrolled by them.

One way to regain perspective is to keep things simple.

HIGH VIBE REFRAME

MY WELL-BEING = OTHERS' WELL-BEING

You are an energy conduit. Happiness wants to be shared. When you feel high vibe, you pass it on. Investing in yourself is an investment in everyone. Sometimes we get stuck in a rut; I've been there. I've felt so uninspired by my life because it felt like a battle instead of a dance. When I feel low, I turn to those low-vibe habits that keep me distracted and focused on what's missing. I keep pushing and doing and running myself down.

HIGH VIBE REFRAME

OVERUSING LOW-VIBE FEELINGS, LIKE GUILT AND REGRET, KEEPS YOU FROM TAKING PRODUCTIVE ACTION.

Gifts, grades, compliments, recognition. Receiving is something we're taught comes from outside of us, but control includes what we give ourselves. Things like compassion, love, patience, and praise are acts we tend to reserve for other people. I have a theory that these various forms of self-compassion are triggered in us through our sense of sight and hearing. It's difficult to show ourselves these acts of kindness because we don't see ourselves from an external perspective. I've found visualization a really powerful ally in being able to turn these behaviors inward. Seeing a younger version of myself or just creating some separation lets me witness my emotions and helps elicit a more loving response. We can feel our pain, sadness, or frustration and respond with the empathy we would show a friend.

One of the things about teaching the High Vibe Habits is that people assume things about me. People are surprised to hear that I also fall prey to low-vibe feelings at times. Part of being human is realizing no matter how experienced we are, we will all still be imperfect. And that means I make mistakes, big ones even. I hold myself to the highest standard with my children. Even there, I do not always set the example I would like to. Not that long ago, I had a moment where I became the exact opposite of what I wanted to model: loud, emotional, and melted down.

Why did this happen?

The answer was my lesson.

It came to me during my apology. I didn't take care of myself; I made no time to decompress, to slow down, to breathe, to recenter. When I'm run down, everyone feels it, and when I'm full, everyone feels it. It's not an excuse for my behavior, it's how I learn to not make the same mistakes.

I microdosed happiness, picked myself up, and turned things around. I apologized, checked in with each of my kids, and even found a win. Imperfection, as ugly as it can look, holds the chance for connection when we accept ourselves instead of judge ourselves.

When I took back control, the High Vibe Habits offered me insight from somewhere deep inside. I don't know if it's intuitive knowledge or universal wisdom. Either way, it supports me and my loved ones. My response to my actions ended up being the example I wanted to set for my children.

It's taken me a long time to feel like making mistakes is acceptable for me as a coach and mother, and it's taken me even longer to feel comfortable sharing them. But, of all the lessons, this is one of the biggies: take good care of yourself when you do well *and* when you fall short.

You will make mistakes. You will be wrong sometimes. But you can say sorry. You can forgive yourself. You can learn. You can hold the lesson close to your heart and still move forward. You can stop judging, comparing, and replaying your lowest moments. Guilt, embarrassment, and self-loathing are not great motivators, but great ruminators that keep us stuck. Continuous low-vibe emotions have us looking backward. Our attempt to feel better requires us to keep revisiting our mistakes. Instead, we can look forward to what we want to be and what we want to create. Guilt isn't resolved when someone else forgives us. It dissolves when we forgive ourselves. Staying unstuck is our greatest challenge and how we evolve. It is the greatest positive ripple effect you can create in the world.

Exploring Blocks

When it comes to control, where might you be building barriers? Let's check out some of the danger zones.

Stability

Controlling things outside of us makes life more predictable. When we are doing things, we know when they get done, how they get done, and how well they get done.

Sometimes we feel like we're the glue that holds it all together. We become Atlas, burdened and stuck.

HIGH VIBE REFRAME

WHAT IF THE LAST THREAD YOU'RE CLINGING TO ISN'T HOLDING YOU UP, BUT HOLDING YOU BACK?

Control is exercising a kind of surrender. Building trust requires uncertainty. Stepping out from under the weight of controlling into the lightness of control can be a relief. If this transition sounds scary, I get it. But when you start to transfer the energy you spend on controlling things around you, you have more energy to spend on shaping the moment that matters—right now. You pay attention to how you're showing up and what you're contributing. That personal progress brings fulfillment into our lives and influences everything and everyone around us. You are a powerful and influential part of your life equation. When you change, you change your life.

Most of us can feel the uptick in our level of frantic energy when we spread ourselves thinly. But the beauty of having a healthy habit that gives us perspective is that it works any time, in any situation. It's a universal solution because it's a lens, not a list. That's why I keep talking about making intentional choices. When we live on purpose, we stay more connected to what we want and are more likely to choose the actions that get us there. You might feel like you don't have choices, and that's partly what clarity helped you start to demystify. There are more options open to us than we can initially see. Control is the same way. We can be so used to making choices that we've always made, or that make other people comfortable, that we forget that there are more options.

Sometimes we are at our last straw, clinging to a final thread. We might be waiting desperately for a new financial situation, or more business. Maybe we feel like we'll lose hope if love or success doesn't come our way soon. Desperation can leave us tightly grasping to what seems like a slim hope. But being high vibe means an alternate perspective presents itself. What if that last thread that you're holding onto isn't holding you up? What if it's holding you back? Control is surrendering to outcomes; it's intentionally snipping that thread that releases us to trust in ourselves and in what lies ahead. Remember, you've survived one hundred percent of your bad days.

When we accept that we have control in life, we are liberated from the enormous weight of other people's choices. The life we build is a collaboration with other people and the Universe. There are things I contribute to, but there are also things for which I am not the sole deciding factor. Accepting the sphere of influence allows us to redirect our thoughts and energy.

It's worth repeating: We have control over ourselves and we influence the rest of our lives. The more self-preparation we do, the more likely we are to experience life positively.

Emotional Math

Valuing your health and happiness requires you to make "sense" of your choice—to see the value in it for other people so you can feel more comfortable making a choice that feels good for you. We run through this kind of calculation before we book that massage, say yes to a night out, or sit down for a break. We find ourselves making excuses and tallying our needs under the "I don't really need this" column, diverting just enough resources our way to stay afloat.

When we are fortunate enough to be in a position to set a thriving goal for ourselves, we also have to redefine and reevaluate what gets prioritized. At this point, our wants might be classified as high-level needs. That extra hour of sleep, reading for pleasure, the gym membership. Just because we can go without those things, doesn't mean we need to. Prioritizing our health and happiness means being willing to value the things that help us create a happy and healthy internal environment. Inconveniencing others is not the same thing as taking from them. Being less available at times might translate to having more available to give. In the end, we choose ourselves so we can keep showing up for others.

Keep this simple math equation in your back pocket: Emotions are information. Listen to your needs. Meet them. Needs can disguise themselves as wants, making them easier to ignore. Use this equation to get clear on what it will take to attain and sustain the life you want.

You can also use this to maintain goal momentum. Seeing something through means doing things we enjoy and that we're good at, and plenty of things that we don't like and probably aren't great at. When we get to the parts that feel like drudgery, our emotions trip the alarm. We hear all the signals that tell us to stop. We feel tired, irritable, and maybe stressed. We're bombarded with low-vibe signals. Just like uncertainty is required for trust, discomfort is a requirement for growth.

I hear the chiming bells and feel irritated. What sounded fairly pleasant when I first set my alarm ring tone sounds like nails on a chalkboard. It's 5:15 a.m. I don't want to get up, but I do. I grab my headphones and tune into my morning meditation. From there I move downstairs, our floorboards creaking, leaving an audible trail of my path to the kitchen. I go through all the motions: tea, chair, computer, write. I do this day in and day out. By 8 a.m., I've essentially squeezed in a full day of work. I'm ready to happily begin the homeschooling day that lies in front of me.

The only way I have been able to stick to this routine through its highs and lows and feel in control is because I acknowledged, but didn't give in to, how I felt when it got hard. I witnessed the fruits of my labor, and it felt good in the end, even if it didn't always feel good in the middle. Creating a joyful space to educate my children requires me to remove as much pressure as possible and have realistic expectations. I've experimented enough with my day to know how much space each pie piece of my life needs to be productive and feel good. Because I've used the reflective habits of curiosity and creativity (both High Vibe Habits), I knew I was creating checkpoints to give myself space to see if this system of operating worked and felt good, or if this was really as exhausting as it felt some days.

Staying the course for long enough allows us to have that fresh perspective, but it helps us in those hard moments when our bodies and minds want to put down the torch. We come to our aid by reminding ourselves that we get to take notice of how we feel but don't have to base our decisions on those feelings, not now anyway. We promise ourselves a time for that.

Visibly tracking your writing progress. Keeping your running shoes next to your bed. Finding an accountability buddy for meditating. Making lunches the night before. Meal prepping on the weekend. There are a boatload of strategies to implement to help us along. They are also part of how we exercise healthy control. They set us up for success. They take the *I have to* and turn them into *I get to*. They give us time to witness our progress. It's a relief to know we don't have to ignore how we feel or let our emotions dictate what we do. All the High Vibe Habits keep things simple and let us feel supported. Chugging along like this has the pleasant benefit of creating those healthy and supportive habits that become second nature. What you want becomes easier to achieve because you paved the way.

MY EMOTIONS DON'T NEED TO DICTATE MY DECISIONS.

Stick to your goals. Create the habits that free you to choose who you want to be. What do you want for yourself? Better health? More patience? Less anger? More compassion? Less stress? Taking that deep breath, checking in with your emotional state, and microdosing happiness gives you the seconds you need to step back and see that there's always more than one door in front of you. You decide which way to go.

I Am

Stuckness, whether it's our thoughts, actions, or inactions, blocks us from feeling like we have agency in our lives. Choosing your state instead of being a product of other people's is what we are looking to create with control. Without creating change for ourselves, our life becomes the same story on repeat. Life can feel draining if the only side you see is what's not there, what's missing. Being inspired by others is great. Looking longingly at a life that feels like it will never be yours is disheartening. We don't find the motivation to go on, to initiate change, if we have lost hope in possibility.

When I first began my writing journey, story after story poured out of me. I am fortunate to be deeply loved and cared for, but my life, like many people's, isn't perfect. The pages became my safe space to share everything I had ever wanted to say. I wrote everything I held in that might hurt someone's feelings, which expressed emotions I had kept tucked away. Unleashing them felt good. So, I kept on. Until I felt empty. The reservoir was tapped. But I had fanned a flame. I had shared my story in a way I never felt I had the permission to. The feelings it drudged up were on the surface now. There was rawness, pain, and tears. I wasn't sure I could go back and read what I had written.

But I did, and what I read surprised me. The collective effect of my written work was not untrue, but it was one-sided. As I reread the stories, it was so clear that this version, this story I had told, was just one side of the story. All the loving and joyful memories flooded back to me. The warmth, love, and happiness of my youth were missing from the pages but not missing from my life. Writing turned out to be a profound experience. I wrote with the mission to help you, and I ended up helping myself along the way.

There's truth to all the versions of our story. But if we're only telling one version, we're only seeing one version. We can't experience what we don't allow ourselves to witness. Life is hard. Life is exhausting. Life is also beautiful. Life is enriching. Life is the story we tell. Chimamanda Ngozi Adichie's TED Talk, *The Danger of a Single Story,* alludes to the idea that one-sided viewpoints cloud our ability to see the multifaceted nature of people. And this also happens with the story we tell ourselves. You are in control of the story you see, the story you tell, and the story you hope to tell.

What do you find yourself saying over and over again? Being high vibe isn't about ignoring any piece of your life. It's about seeing *all* the pieces. Creating a complete picture for yourself on purpose. Believing that we can't change, or our lives can't change, denies us the truth—change is possible. When we feel like we're carried along by the wind, we're at its mercy. Whether we're walking on eggshells in our homes, or we get knocked down when other people take things out on us, we live reactively instead of proactively. Having a clear destination lets us choose our steps, dancing our way to our desires.

Control Versus Controlling

If you haven't practiced tuning into the nuance between these two concepts, it can be a little tricky. Pausing to observe your motivation helps to identify fear-based actions from high vibe ones. Fear drives us towards things like doubt, worry, distrust, impatience, and rigidity. It shifts our focus from the present to the future (usually worrying about an outcome).

To gain access to the habit of control, we have to know how to tell it apart from its less helpful look-alike: controlling. If it originates within you, that's the domain of control. It's pretty simple, but easy to forget, thanks to distracted lifestyle habits that keep us too busy to tell the difference sometimes. We lose control when external factors define and guide our internal values and actions. We give up our power.

Let's look at the three things we try to control: people, outcomes, and time.

Controlling affects stress levels, relationships, and even goal setting. Anything that contributes to chronic stress alters our well-being. We get better at relating to others as we get better at understanding ourselves.

Doing work that others are capable of doing can create a lifelong dependence. That's a situation from which we can't remove ourselves because they didn't develop the skills to support themselves. Instead of offering scaffolding to build themselves up, we put them on our shoulders. And while it might create temporary good feelings, it doesn't maintain high vibrational states because as we exert our thoughts, opinions, and will upon others, we feel better, but they often feel squashed.

We can lead people. We can teach people. We can do things for other people— just not all the time. Other people will always make decisions we wouldn't, have ideas we don't have and want to attempt things we wouldn't. One of the things we have to unlearn is the belief that control is something we exert outside of ourselves. When we redirect that energy within, we are better at influencing the outcomes we want while expending less energy. We also begin to support those around us without needing to be their answer.

You could look at control as a mindfulness practice. You are doing what you can right now to influence a future moment. When you manage your actions, you positively influence outcomes. Holding onto your vision is important but so is being able to toggle back to the present so you can be intentional and impactful. Improving prioritization skills and emotional efficiency impacts how you experience time. Removing the barriers to a high-vibe life, coupled with time-saving strategies, helps you steer clear of your natural negative and ruminating tendencies.

Sometimes, we exert control because we believe no one else will do the job as well as us. But other times it's the very real lack of supportive infrastructure in our homes, families, and societies that leaves us with a huge mental load. Top that off with the lessons we learn from the school of learned deprivation, and controlling might feel like the only option. As a survival mechanism, it's what we cling to in order to keep ourselves afloat. But it rarely makes us feel supported, which is what we need to feel to expand our lives.

A lot of our controlling energy comes from our desire to see ourselves or those around us flourish, rather than feel pain. But a good intention doesn't change the truth that we are each already in control of ourselves. There's liberation in knowing that each of us gets this power so that none of us needs to be responsible for someone else's life.

Control is exhilarating because it gives us the security we're looking for. No more of that roller coaster feeling. When we know we know who we are and what we want, the control we practice on ourselves translates to confidence. Others pick up on that sure-footedness and follow suit. My truth becomes my reality. When I love myself, I better attract loving relationships. When I believe in myself, more people believe in me. When I respect myself, others are more respectful of me. I've seen this over and over

again in my own life and my clients' lives—
and it's not magic. Our beliefs change our
thoughts, which changes what we do. There's
always a connection between thoughts and
actions.

What If

The biggest blocks to regaining control
are our unproductive thoughts. They leave us
overwhelmed, stressed, exhausted, and
overthinking things. Sitting with your
feelings, logic, and intuition are ways to
gather information. But many times, after we
gather, we stew. The internal conflict
between what feels right versus easy versus
expected makes us feel indecisive. Not
wanting to make a wrong choice leads us to
spend more time with negative scenarios
than possible positive ones.

We need to shift into action mode. I once
heard Tony Robbins explain fear and faith as
essentially the same thing. Both, he said, are
belief in what *hasn't* happened yet. We tend
to feel like our fears are a more honest
appraisal of what lies ahead. Faith, or trust,
can feel like a positive Pollyanna thought
somehow ignoring reality. I believe there's a

place for all our emotions. Recognizing we hold fear at any level means we have the chance to harvest information. Trusting in ourselves requires confidence (the next habit we'll cover), but that confidence comes in part from taking control of our thoughts.

It's important to learn that our first thought isn't necessarily a true thought. I know how much weight we can give that first voice that chimes in, but it's usually the most reactive, fear-based one. The likelihood of it being negative tends to make it feel safer to believe. Remember, one job of fear is to help us avoid pain. Control sometimes means not believing everything you tell yourself. Recognizing a reactive thought versus a more thoughtfully weighted one is an act of control.

Thinking requires a great deal more energy than doing. Thoughts are complex and can be drawn out far into the future based purely on our imaginations. At this point, we can create many scenarios without feeling any better because we're recycling what's already inside our minds. What we do in the present moment, and the actions we take, offers us new information because once we do something, we've changed what we've got to work with. It's practice for distinguishing a perceived fear from an actual threat.

Fear

You've probably noticed a common underlying thread as we've explored how we block our joy: fear is the main culprit here. We create a scenario in our minds where we fear being deprived of basic needs like security, connection, or love. This fear taps into a primal instinct of ours—avoid pain. Interdependence is one reason for our existence today. It's why what other people think is such a big deal. Another big portion of our evolutionary success is due to our ability to think up dangerous scenarios so we can avoid them.

Uncertainty feeds the perceived fears in our heads. When fears are real, rumination often makes them feel disproportionate. Ask yourself, *what would happen if I...?* Try filling in the blank with your fear. This is a really powerful question to ask yourself because fear of the unknown often blinds us from our options.

Have you ever noticed how worst-case scenarios somehow seem more plausible than best-case ones? Our minds are great at playing this what-if game. And these situations are usually the first things to pop into our heads. My advice? Don't believe everything you tell yourself. Initial thoughts can take a while to rewire. Here's a new what-if game for you. What would you do if happiness was in your control? What if you actually did the thing that made you happy?

What stops you from making a decision? Which ones feel hard? What would actually happen if you stopped saying yes to the extra stuff at work? Do you fear people won't like you or think you're not a team player? What if you stopped cleaning up after your kids or partner? Would your house turn into a pigsty? And if you stopped agreeing to volunteer at school? Would people think you're not a dedicated mother? Do your questions lead you to wonder what other people think or how to achieve what you want?

If control comes from us, so can the feeling of being out of control. Words, spoken or thought, are powerful. The language we choose can tether us to an experience we don't want. They are a self-created block. Starting sentences with *I am, I'm not, I can't,* and *I don't* are indicators of where we lie on the spectrum of have and lack.

Words are powerful tools for self-oppression. What we say out loud and in our heads gets in the way of our success. Knowing this can also be an easy way to free ourselves. New words create new landscapes for us. If I wake up and think, "I have to" I feel like I'm slogging through my day. If I wake up and say, "I get to" I remember that my lifestyle requires effort, but it moves me towards my goals. It's language that can shift you from seeing your life in terms of costs to seeing it in terms of investments.

Not too long ago, life presented me with a new opportunity to evolve. Every September seems to be full of transitions and all the challenges that go along with them. Last fall, I had a really crazy several weeks. To top off the new schedules, checkups, meetings, classes, and playdates, I'd been solo parenting for almost two weeks. At the end of the first week, I could feel my stress levels settling at an undesirably high baseline. The second week started feeling overwhelming before it even began. When I couldn't kick the stress, I knew something had to change.

First, I changed my language. I stopped saying how overwhelmed I was and how busy and crazy everything was going to be. Thinking is always more exhausting than doing, I reminded myself. I chose to have a more abundant approach. How much fun was I going to have with the kids? This was my chance to fill in for Dad, which meant I got to do some fun stuff too! (Thanks to curiosity and creativity!) I prioritized feeling good and having fun. I realized it's possible to be a high-achieving, responsible adult *and* feel good. (I need to hang that on my refrigerator.)

I found as many opportunities to say yes as I could. That was unusual for me. I also uncovered a belief I didn't realize I had. As a mother, I've felt responsible for the boring to-dos and let my partner get most of the fun stuff. He likes ice cream, lazy weekends, and movie nights—so do I. But I've always wondered if I chose those things, who votes for vegetables, a good night's sleep, and the must-dos that fall on a weekend? My husband contributes around our household, but when he's around I often find myself needing to be the weight that keeps our scales from tipping.

As soon as I had this thought, I wondered. . . *tipping into what?* What am I actually afraid is going to happen?

Asking myself this question awakened me to my perceived fears, another reminder that what we fear isn't a guarantee that it will happen. I couldn't help but notice my story of achieving and deprivation. How can we say yes, have tons of fun, and accomplish our goals? Experimentation is part of the process, but so is possibility.

During those two weeks, the kids and I accomplished all our work (school, classes, book writing, meetings, errands, meals, dishes, house cleaning, laundry, and groceries. . .) and had play dates, a sushi lunch, a mac-and-cheese movie night, cuddly reading time, and video games. Was I tired? Yes. Happy to have my husband home? Yes. But I went from feeling like I needed to survive this time to enjoying it, something I didn't know was possible until I took control. Whatever you're afraid of losing, a clean house, your sanity, community, family, status, or image, it doesn't have to be a given.

The magic was noticing how I felt. Only then could I take control, swoop in, and choose something different. I was able to step back, get a big-picture view, and then find effective solutions that felt good. My overwhelm turned into enjoyment when I implemented my High Vibe Habits.

The brain's purpose is to seek pleasure but also to avoid pain. A life avoiding pain is not the same as a life following your joy. Perspective matters. What you believe matters. Understanding you can change what you believe and knowing how to do it with the High Vibe Habits offers you that broad sense of security you seek. We become our safety net knowing we aren't just equipped for a few situations, but for whatever comes our way.

Goal Setting + Achievement

My home environment used to stress me out a lot. I hated how untidy the house was. I spent a lot of energy managing the house and the little people that made it that way. It stressed all of us out! When I assessed my actual needs and feelings, I found a way to find more peace and less work. I accepted the stage I was in—a mother of two young kids. I accepted that I needed my home space, which was also my workplace, to meet a certain level of organization, but that level wasn't as tidy as my original goal. Lowering my standard of a magazine-perfect home raised my quality of life. Fashion and function can intersect, and so can expectation and reality. It frees up a ton of mental and physical energy and time.

Charles Cooley said, "I am not who you think I am; I am not who I think I am; I am who I think you think I am." As we seek to connect, be liked, and feel valued within our communities, our fears often stop us from seeing our choices and taking action because of the imagined consequences. This negative thought pattern brings on an onslaught of feelings. You've heard me say that feelings and emotions offer us information. When we stew in those scary or anxious thoughts, it's usually enough to prevent our ideas and dreams from being realized. Action is an essential element in bringing what lies within us out of us.

October 2022 marked the first anniversary of my newsletter and blog. It was once a wild idea filled with questions about how I was going to accomplish it. Writing weekly content wasn't something I'd ever done, and it seemed enormously daunting. The voices in my head chimed in: *What could I possibly say? What would my readers want to hear every single week? Who would listen?*

But I did it anyway.

Here's the thing I want to remind you. Every large, impossible, daring, audacious thing you desire can be broken down into small, bite-sized, manageable steps. Uncertainty in ourselves and the process can easily stop us. So, let the fact that you want something be the first step in trusting that you will create it. This trust is simply you committing to yourself that you're all in.

I didn't sit down that first day and write fifty-two letters. I devoted a little time every week to sharing my experiences with my audience. I took a small step every week — just one letter to them.

It's been a journey for me. I've gone from writing the task in my planner to using the idea of these letters as my motivation to stay tuned in to my feelings and my life, and trust that there is always a lesson that will present itself to me. All I need to do is be ready to receive.

I've heard a lot of people refer to it as a "divine download." Sounds beautiful, doesn't it? When you get clarity about what you want in your life, are open to hearing it, and are courageous enough to make it come true.

Be your dreamcatcher. It's that last step that gets us. Control doesn't mean you're assured of certain victory in the end, it means choosing to see every step forward as a victory. We can make things happen even if we don't initially know how. Simply by deciding we will, we will find the way. Certainly, there are times when it hasn't all worked, but it's never a loss. We keep growing because we keep going. Each intentional choice is a step. Exercising control is moving ourselves up the mountain that gives us a fresh perspective.

A friend forwarded me this email once. It said:

How to achieve a vision:

1. Know your desired outcome.

2. Not know how you'll pull it off.
3. Proceed anyway.

When you move, I move — *The Universe*.

I have no doubt you know one thing you want. Start today. If it feels overwhelming, reverse engineer it until it's just one doable thing. Take that one small step. Again. And again. And again.

Sitting in discomfort can show us where we stop trusting ourselves. This clarity is one of the biggest gifts because it means how we feel doesn't have to affect what we do. We get to stop being overwhelmed and start moving ourselves. Action leads to new information. Inaction leads to the same thoughts that usually produce the same results. The upcoming C's—confidence, curiosity, and creativity—will show you how to support this action. Replace habits of anger, yelling, procrastination, rumination, and self-doubt. Let empathy, creativity, love, confidence, and courage be the habits that lead you onward and upward.

Every huge decision you'll ever make breaks down into a series of small acts. Many things are possible. A great place to start is in valuing the little pieces of the puzzle. Small consistent steps create vast amounts of change. My blogging journey, writing this book, eating healthy, moving my body—all these are a series of small, consistent steps I take that lead me closer and closer to a happy and healthy life.

There's a last block I want to mention: worthiness or feeling enough. Though it's also fear-based, it's worth talking about. A lot of us have very little self-empathy. We pride ourselves on high-quality results and judge ourselves and others because we believe it's what leads to success. Having standards doesn't require a negative lens. Fear is a motivator, but there are other more constructive approaches. Pessimism and negative self-talk may have been effective tools in the past, this encourages us to keep implementing them, but we suffer from them and so does our end goal of thriving.

It's possible to link achievement with joy and become an inspired achiever, rather than a deprived one. Being an achiever means being your best. Each C contributes to this end. Control leads you to aligned action— that's energy not just spent, but invested, towards a goal. Each C lets you set the bar high but leaves space for you to feel positive, expansive, powerful, and impactful. Earning the external indicators of success doesn't automatically make us feel like we're enough. We can grant ourselves this kindness. Imperfection doesn't make you flawed; it makes you human. We may be wired to keep doing whatever it is we've been doing, but we're also wired to adapt and evolve.

Belonging

Claim your squatter's rights. You probably know this, but in many places around the world, if you live in a place long enough you get the right to live there. Hopefully, you haven't had to deal with this issue before, but I invite you to try this reframe.

On your way to living a high-vibe life, it can be easy to succumb to the old habits that keep you low. At either end of the vibrational spectrum, our emotional state acts like a whirlpool. It draws us in, keeping us feeling either good or poorly. Maybe you make lots of decisions and it's tiring. Maybe you've let other people decide things for you. There's a way to feel in control with more ease and less stress. If I wasn't worried about the outcome, what would I do? Where would I turn my attention? There's plenty to focus on where you are and plenty to worry about where you aren't. In the beginning, all things feel unfamiliar and unlike us. It's like a new haircut—at first, we don't recognize ourselves, but with time we identify with the new image.

While you practice your High Vibe Habits, imagine you're the squatter. The longer you spend in that high vibe "home" the more right you feel you have to be there. No matter how many times you get kicked out, keep showing up. You're doing big work to change a belief system. The newness or discomfort you feel isn't a sign you don't belong; it's a sign you're growing.

Don't be a stranger to the life you want. You are worth it. And the high-vibe world is your home. It can't feel that way if you don't spend time there. No matter how many times you have to choose your way back into the driver's seat in life, no matter how many times you have to pull yourself out of a low-vibe zone, just keep showing up.

There are a lot of things that can get us down. Bad things happen daily. There's always someone having a tough day, ready to take their stress out on someone else.

Learning to be the light lets us see the light in others. Starting with ourselves, we make the world a brighter place.

How do you start? It's a simple two-step process.

Ask, how do I feel right now? And *listen*. The answer matters because you matter.

Offer yourself what you need. It could be rest, movement, connection, joy, fun, nourishment, silence, or laughter. Make space for you.

This chapter's breakdown:

CONTROL **encourages**:
agency, growth mindset, perseverance, resilience, goal actualization, self-preparedness, happiness, health, acceptance, patience, responsiveness, self-compassion, excellence, fulfillment, solution-oriented mindset, motivation, empathy, peace

---

CONTROL **eliminates**:
perfectionism, procrastination, feeling responsible for other people's behaviors or emotions, overwhelm, indecision, reactiveness, internal conflict, exhaustion, hustle culture, fear-based overthinking, external pressure, regret, guilt, judgment

---

EXERCISES + INSIGHTS

This is your judgment-free zone reminder!

Access to control comes through clarity. Being aware of how you feel, what you think, and how you show up, lets you see why you are or aren't having the life experience you want. If I want to prioritize my health and happiness, I get to find a way to choose it while I'm living my life. It's not an end product, it's a path.

I've exposed you to the habits in a particular order. You will use them each consecutively and you'll use them in layers. But here's what your high-vibe habits look like so far:

- Clarity first. Recognize that you're not feeling good and remember the goal is to feel better.

- Control is what I am going to do to move in that direction. Pause and microdose happiness. Choose to do something about it. (Like that drop-by-drop ink imagery, we choose which ink dropper to use, to feel good or not.)

If you're on a constructive path, great! If not, follow these stepping stones. Life is a series of the act of choosing again. Whether it's a feeling, thought, or a course of action—you decide if you'll stay on that path or head in another direction. I invite you to implement control in each of the realms of your life: work, finances, love, dreams, goals, to-dos, and responsibilities.

Control is the dance you do with life and everyone in it. Here are some exercises to help you through each of the areas you get to practice this habit.

Release

Control is also about receiving. You can learn to intentionally create a more relaxed internal environment for yourself. But to do that, you need to know:

- How do I feel right now?
- How do I want to feel?
- What thoughts are taking me out of my high-vibe zone?

You don't need to stew in your feelings to acknowledge them. Witnessing your state can be a quick process. Practice makes deep connections. Once you gain the knowledge those feelings offer you, you get to learn to let them go as you take action in this control habit. Use these prompts to reflect in your journal. The goal is to eventually be able to do this mentally throughout your day.

NOTES

Body Scan

Your body is telling you things all the time. Learn how to harvest that information. Create specific times when you will check in with your body. By attaching them to what's already a part of your life, it can feel easier to maintain this habit. It could be when your alarm goes off; before you stop for lunch or right after; during your commute; or before you turn in for the evening. Setting aside regular times to check in creates a strong internal connection, which is the compass that guides you toward high-vibe states.

- Closing your eyes, start at the top of your head and see how your body feels. Is there any discomfort or tension?
- Stay in any of those places and take an extra moment to breathe into those tense areas, helping them relax.
- Notice the thoughts that might be contributing to your tension.

NOTES

Bookends

Cycles exist all around us and within us. This practice is about learning how to consciously create that feeling of productivity and presence through flow. Flow is found more easily when we aren't depleted. Bookends are purposeful breaks in your day to make sure you're checking your personal fuel gauge. Finding flow within each day helps us avoid that go-go-go-crash negative model. Resting is also productive and contributes to long-term success.

Cycling between blocks of productivity and rest keeps my energy and creative juices flowing. The outcome leads to more fulfillment because it sets me up to be productive and present. Setting aside regular times to check in creates a strong internal connection, which is the compass that guides us toward high-vibe states.

This act is especially individualized due to each person's personality and their work environment. The challenge is to honor your individual pace when those around you function differently. Built in pauses have made me more productive and fulfilled.

NOTES

Creating Routines

The point is to first investigate what might be weighing on you. What's difficult for you to do that you would like to do? Does shutting off your work thoughts to enjoy family dinner feel hard? Do you feel rushed or forgetful in the morning? This is an exercise to identify where you need support and how to automate it a bit.

What might this look like?

- **A.M. routine:** meditate, morning hygiene, breakfast
- **Start workday:** cup of tea, review prioritized list for the day
- **End workday:** close all work-related windows on my computer, write my prioritized list

for the following day, review
remaining personal tasks
- **P.M. routine:** put away all devices,
  wind down routine with my
  children and bedtime, read

Other things to consider: lighting a
candle, working out, walking, socializing, a
favorite show, music, dance, hobbies, etc.

Your routine will be unique to you. Just
remember this is not about distracting you
from life but about experiencing it.

Changing how we see changes *what* we
see. Live on purpose. I'm inviting you to think
about life not just in terms of what you want to
produce and create, but what you want to
experience.

It often only takes a little perspective to
find joy in the life you've built. I have devoted
many years to pursuing my passions, both
personal and professional. Yet, I was unable to
feel fulfilled by my choices because I wasn't
able to receive. I was living for a perfect future,
forgetting to cherish the experience that is life.
Learning to take back control of my life has
brought me more than I could have imagined.

Let these habits and exercises guide you to
find your unique values and lifestyle. Leave

behind any judgment of what you "should" want or do. Embrace the journey inwards. Reap the rewards everywhere. Set aside any feelings of scarcity. If you live and work from a place of fear (judgment, guilt, regret, or shame), your only option is to do more of the same. Why not arm yourself with the mindset and skill set of constructive habits and become the solution? You are the author of your own story.

The life you want is found through intentional living. Making conscious choices means you actively choose one thing over another. That act of choice, when aligned with our values, brings fulfillment and empowerment. Time gets spent minute by minute, choice by choice. If you don't choose how to spend your time and energy, someone else will.

NOTES

For more Control exercises, visit www.nithyakaria.com/highvibebook.

66

Almost every successful person begins with two beliefs:
the future can be better than the present,
and I have the power to make it so.

— *David Brooks*

FIVE

CONFIDENCE

She's born with it.

Tell me I'm not the only one who's seen a put-together, confident person and thought for sure, they must've been born that way.

In high school, it was the cool kids. In college, I admired the social butterflies. Later, it would be colleagues who spoke up. Each one of those people seemed to possess this no-fear aura. And I wanted it.

I wanted it the way you might want an amazing leather jacket in a boutique window. I dreamt about it. I tried it on. But I didn't buy it for the longest time. *Who was I to go around valuing myself and my ideas?* It seemed too good for me.

I was stuck in that distracted state of comparison and judgment that had me doubting myself. My focus was on everything I wasn't. While I could feel confident in certain situations, there were still so many moments when I didn't feel comfortable in my skin. Life felt like a performance, and I wasn't always sure I was playing the part right.

She's special. I'm not. We are so good at making ourselves separate from everyone else, especially when it comes to our "faults." The things we wish we were or wish we had, are as un-destined for us as they are inevitable for someone else. We talked about those powerful words, *I am*, in the last chapters and how we tell ourselves a story: I can't change this part of me or this part of my life. We admire other people for their calm, their cool, their strength, and their attitude. And then we take a look in the mirror and see our shortcomings. We resign ourselves to the belief that we are what we are. But I'll bet you're great at something. Do you see that part of yourself? Do you see what you've overcome, created, sustained, and managed? It's time to transform these old habits of comparison, judgement, and jealousy into inspiration. Look around. What you see isn't a sign of what you aren't, it's a sign of what's possible.

I got so used to seeing myself a certain way, that I forgot that my abilities weren't static. I know why too. Low vibe thinking requires us to prove ourselves. I would put myself in "test" situations and I wouldn't "pass." I couldn't live up to my unrealistic expectations. I let that be my confirmation of the same old story: *I'm not___.* But the more I believed that I could grow confidence, the more permission I gave myself to experiment with a different approach. Small steps. They weren't changing me overnight, but they were changing me over time.

I looked through a new lens. I found ways to use my strengths in places where I felt uncomfortable. In large groups, my goal became to meet two new people and connect with them beyond the surface-level discussions. I recognized what I wasn't—an entertainer. I also knew what I was—curious and a great listener. Drawing on pieces of who I already was became my way of creating a sense of comfort within me so I could show up confidently in previously uncomfortable situations.

Watching my growth was the confirmation that I could evolve. Transferring my focus from imperfection to growth helped remove the pedestal model in my life. You know that feeling where you set others up high because they're better? It's a model where we see the lack between us and others—a distance so great we resign ourselves to not being enough. If you're not preset with a confidence level, what does that mean for you? Confidence isn't handed to you; it's a gift you give yourself.

Once I began to see that I wasn't completely flawed and everyone else wasn't completely perfect, I began trying to figure out how to cultivate my confidence. It's true that I'm never going to be the person I admire. But I am going to be my version of what I want to be. Our interpretation and unique application of skills are our strengths. It's the wabi-sabi approach. That's a Japanese concept that believes in the uniqueness of imperfection as beauty, not blemish.

Confidence is the third High Vibe Habit. I mentioned three phases to maintaining a high-vibe path: plan (clarity), do (control), and review. We're entering some new territory in this chapter. It straddles the line between doing and reviewing. Confidence is applied in a forward direction, helping you take action, and as a reflective habit as you look back. The High Vibe Habits are layering habits. I've tried to break them into singular lessons, but the goal is to put them all together and have access to each habit at any time. Our minds flow between these phases at a rapid speed. Practicing the High Vibe Habits on repeat is how we quickly find our way back to constructive living when we veer off the path. As habits, they'll all be running in the background together to help you prioritize your health and happiness.

Why does this C feel like such a big deal? I don't know a single person who wouldn't want it. We want confidence because it feels so good. Being yourself always does. Operating from a space of comfort makes us feel safe and worthy. Many of us spend so much time not feeling comfortable in our skin. Presenting ourselves as put-together, young, beautiful, smart, successful, or happy can feel like a game of dress-up as we hide behind a made-up façade. Confidence is accepting who we are, not finding ways to cover ourselves up.

It's great to feel good at something, but even better to feel good about yourself. The kind of confidence that permeates your whole being. The kind that isn't dependent on the task. It's knowing that you are enough and are resourceful enough for what is called for. It's a complete and true belief in yourself. It's about how you see your failures, your worth, and your place.

HIGH VIBE REFRAME

YOU CREATE MEANING.

Growth Mindset

There's a long list of traits that contribute to our overall sense of fullness. But it isn't mastery alone that allows us to show up powerfully. We benefit from a growth mindset. We stop questioning our value. We accept that we learn even if we "lose," which shifts our perception to value process instead of only outcome. Confidence is also about resourcefulness. We get to ask new questions. *What does this situation need and how can I show up with this?* (These questions reflect the next two habits: curiosity and creativity.)

The fear I hear over and over again is, "If I don't ___, people will do/think ___." But I think an additionally painful part of this line of thinking is the fear that we'll offer ourselves proof that we aren't enough. I'm not: *hardworking. . . worthy. . . capable. . . intelligent. . . beautiful. . . lovable.* It's our subconscious saying, *I told you*, and that deals a big blow.

Okay, so we all want confidence, but what's happening when we don't have enough of it? Why is it important to actively cultivate? If confidence comes from comfort, then not having it places you in a zone of discomfort. That perceived "pain" shifts your brain into a fear-based stress mode. Your brain on fear has different thoughts, makes different choices, and alters potential outcomes. What does all that mean? You show up differently. Newness lends itself to discomfort. Confidence in yourself lets you feel more comfortable being uncomfortable. You might be able to reduce the size of your discomfort zone. Creating that safe space within you irrespective of what happens around you lets you have consistent access to your higher-level thinking.

Confidence is fostered through clarity and control when used reflectively. It impacts our relationships, work, and hopes. It changes what we do. Insecurity can come from believing she has something or is something, I'm not. I've heard everything from stamina, beauty, luck, energy, money, experience, or confidence as areas in which women compare themselves. That separation of ourselves from everyone else has us seeing ourselves through a distorted lens and making decisions from where we *think* we are instead of where we are. This can blind us from improving and deny us the progress we've made.

In each High Vibe C, you get to practice identifying and deconstructing your old habits. Finding where you are creating resistance to what you want works because you're not just releasing the blocks, you're replacing the habits that create them. Imagine trying to stop eating a ritual late-night snack by only saying that you would stop. What would happen when that reflex kicked in if you didn't have another way to handle the habit? Every time you don't make that aligned choice, you reinforce the idea of what you "knew" all along: I can't create change. But what happens when you practice your High Vibe Habits?

A new journey begins. You seek clarity to know why you started snacking in the first place. Comfort? Hunger? Entertainment? Then you get to choose an alternative. Keep yourself busy. Stop buying those tempting snacks. Get to bed earlier. Snack earlier in the day. Eat a smaller snack and wean yourself. This is where you implement a strategy and see what works for you. Confidence can be mined after each positive decision. It can also be applied in the moment.

As you reach for that bag of chips, pause. Live on purpose. You're giving up the chips now, but what does the future you gain? The smallest step in the direction of your goal is enough to add a tally mark under your "I can" column.

Let's look at confidence under a microscope. Confidence, according to Merriam-Webster, is a feeling of trust or belief. Trust and belief. *It matters what you believe*. This is the foundational idea we began with back in Chapter One. Remember that beliefs are thoughts and ideas that you accept as truth. They are malleable because you create them. That's huge. That means you can stop wishing and start working towards what you want.

Confidence feels good. That "good" feeling is freedom. Freedom to create the life you want. Freedom from living by other people's expectations. Experiencing a truly confident moment in life is so energizing because it fills you with so many positive emotions. It frees you to have a deeper experience because you're focused on what's happening outside of you instead of being distracted by what's happening inside of you. Accomplishing things expands our comfort zone. It's proof of agency. When we aren't busy managing the fear and discomfort within, we are available to see new things, learn new things, and grow. Growth is an accomplishment and builds our confidence. Even if we stumble through something, we get through it. What doesn't break us, builds us. Every day is potential fuel for your confidence fire.

Data Versus Story

What would be possible if you set aside fear? What would you want? What would you do? Imagine how different your life would be. What would you accomplish and what would you desire? It might change the partner you're with, the job you have, the size of your bank account, or your aspirations.

The world would be a very different place if we found more confidence. Sounds a bit dramatic, but the reality is that we change our trajectory, degree by degree, with every single choice we make. It all adds up and lands us in a very different place.

Have you ever had a question or idea, but were intimidated by the people around you and stayed quiet? The belief that you shouldn't contribute or aren't supposed to? Or that your voice might even be unwanted? We learn early on that questions might be judged, and authority doesn't always like to be questioned. You've probably either felt the sting of embarrassment for asking a "dumb" question or witnessed it happen to someone else. We avoid pain by staying quiet. Instead of experiencing our voice as a powerful contribution, we see it as a way to bring on unnecessary discomfort. Our fear dial gets turned up.

We are always learning. Believing that we should only contribute after we know all the answers is one way to hold ourselves back. I'm not saying you have to jump into every conversation, but I'll bet that most of us have a question that went unanswered or an idea that we never shared. Contribution is not exclusively top-down. Perspective can come from any direction and is a powerful vehicle for growth.

There's study after study where scientists have made confidence, or the lack of it, tangible. It shows up in our words, in our silence, in our asks, and our attempts. These documented comparisons between men and women show how often our self-perception changes what we do. It's not asking for a raise, not applying for a promotion, not questioning authority, or not believing in our ability even when we do take action. Evidence has been collected showing that women executing a task or test performed equally as well as their male counterparts, even though they didn't believe they were as qualified.[12] Disbelief in our capability often

---

[12] Kay, Katty and Shipman, Claire. "The Confidence Gap". *The Atlantic.* May 2014 Issue. https://www.theatlantic.com/magazine/archive/2014/05/the-confidence-gap/359815/

lives only in our minds. The ever-growing data indicating the very real impact of lower confidence isn't meant to be deflating or guilt-inducing. I hope that it diminishes your fear and inspires you to act so we bolster the evidence that says we can do hard things. Confidence contributes to our competence thanks to the availability of integral thinking skills that contribute to our breadth of knowledge, our recall, and the opportunities we create to apply that knowledge.

That's the data, but what's the story? Scientists are always performing studies and creating statistics. Statistics are made up of individual stories. We don't always relate to a number or percentage, but we can relate to a feeling and a situation. I'm not claiming that gender inequality in the workplace is resolved with a boost to women's confidence—there's work to be done by everyone. In the workplace, the deck is stacked against us with men who are more likely to be hired for their potential and women for their track record[13]. But this conditioning begins from the earliest years.

---

[13] "*Genius.*" Joanna Barsh (Ft. Lareina Yee) – Unlocking the Full Potential of Women in the US Economy,"
n.d. https://genius.com/Joanna-barsh-unlocking-the-full-potential-of-women-in-the-us-economy-annotated.

Women more frequently feel like they need to prove their competence and worth and ask for validation or permission for what they want because we've been taught to. Most of these disparity studies take place at work, but many of these traits follow us home.

This book doesn't tackle all the greater work that needs to be done to create a more equitable society; it does help you obliterate the obstacles that inequity planted within you. The one you might be nurturing instead of dismantling. There's always a part of the story we can't control: what other people see in us or think about us. The part we can always work on is what we believe about ourselves. Confidence isn't about how others see you, but how you see yourself.

The story, or cost, of lower confidence levels, is written everywhere. It's your friend not willing to cut herself a little slack. It's your mom accepting less than she deserves. It's your sister not asking for what she's worth. It's your coworker doing extra work in the office for free. It's the girl at the check-out counter not asking for the respect she's due.

This lower self-perception is changing lives and societies. It makes us more vulnerable because we make less money, have less influence, and take on a heavy mental and physical load without adequate support. It also makes us an easy target because we already believe we might be the problem. The reason something didn't go successfully. The reason we don't look the way we want. The reason other people make poor choices. Our beliefs are changing the landscape in which we live.

Growth is a limitless, expansive state. Like an inventor endlessly tinkering to improve her work, we can see in terms of improvement instead of lack. Searching for and working on ourselves can become joyful. Confident or not, be open to any blocks you might be utilizing. You're not a number, but you contribute to a bigger picture. Don't let your old story write your ongoing one.

Confidence might show up very clearly in some areas of your life and fuzzier in others. Belief can fluctuate between environments like work and home, between people like spouses and siblings, or in specific situations like one-on-one conversations and group gatherings. Invest in creating more emotional balance for yourself through confidence-building work. Dedicating time to a practice of self-clarity and connection leads to acceptance of what you have and what you can strengthen. It's getting to know your unique superpowers. It's redefining terms for yourself. It's supporting yourself.

Exploring Blocks

We began with self-clarity because when we have limiting beliefs like "my work is my worth," we find ourselves in competition with others and focused on goals, but missing the opportunity to measure our growth. It's *how have I compared against her* instead of asking how much *I have I grown*. Any shift that lets us see our progress grows our confidence.

I understand that competitive environments exist. There are many events where we are chosen because of the skill we display on paper, on a court, or with clients. But how many times do we show up with the same mindset when we're *not* competing?

Part of our very nature, our basic need, is connection. In today's modern world, if you're not intentional, it can easily turn into comparison and competition. Our need to find a place to fit in within a hierarchy of our own making leaves most of us feeling deflated (more distracted living).

You're not here to prove your worth to anyone. You're here to live your purpose— whatever that looks like for you. You don't need to prove to anyone you're a better boss, mother, employee, wife, or daughter. I invite you to value the journey of uncovering the best version of yourself and be open to evolving.

The good news is that we can connect with people without needing to be better or worse. What kind of confidence would you have if you knew you were enough? We can choose to live constructively and build ourselves and others up. President John F. Kennedy's words have popped up on my radar a few times while writing this chapter: "A rising tide lifts all boats." That's constructive living. Working on feeling good yourself, allowing that to let you see the good around you, and then going on to create a better world. That's a cycle worth repeating.

Comfort To Discomfort

Confidence arises from permission to be yourself and finding value in yourself. You pour into confidence and let it pour back into you. It's a more natural state than you think. When you break it down, it's a state of comfort from being yourself. We probably spend more time in this state than we realize because we aren't used to recognizing our comfort as confidence. We can learn to see our strengths in these moments to help us see what we're leaving behind in less comfortable situations. Do people who know you well see your kindness or wit? Do they see your creativity? Witness your ingenuity? Admire your drive?

HIGH VIBE REFRAME

COMFORT MAKES US FEEL
CONFIDENT BUT DISCOMFORT
GROWS CONFIDENCE.

Our bodies are great at identifying uncomfortable situations. Conversations, situations, and unpredictable events can trigger sweaty palms, butterflies, tight muscles, or a dry throat. Use the information. See where you can draw on strengths you previously didn't access.

You want to be your own safe space. I mentioned this idea when I talked about those three rings of external pressure. Our responsibility as adults is to find an awareness that we can offer ourselves the safety we seek. This is what allows us to grow. Getting comfortable with being uncomfortable is also an important part of life. Fearful thoughts can be a sign that we are nearing expansion. Like the butterfly exiting her cocoon, struggle induces growth. The clarity we can offer ourselves is the distinction between pain and discomfort. Fear stimulates our instinct for pain aversion. But if we can see through the lens of discomfort instead, we evolve.

To have new thoughts, we need new information. Letting our fearful thoughts control our actions compromises our vision. Challenges, effort, and discomfort are part of what creates the joy, sense of accomplishment, and confidence we gain from follow-through. The tough days you've survived are behind you. Let that be evidence that what you need is already within you. Feel secure. The answer isn't outside, it's inside you. The experiences you have are what help draw them out.

The Squeaky Wheel

Courage and fear are related. You and I have a baseline relationship of courage and fear, our current state of mental fitness. Most of us are used to tackling this by building up our courage and preparing ourselves to climb the mountain of fear. But what about a reverse lens to turn the mountain into a molehill? Increasing our courage (see Option 1 below) or diminishing our fear (see Option 2) produces the desired feel-good result we're looking for—confidence.

Courage can be hard to come by at times, so I offer you the High Vibe Habits to have a chance to practice Option 2 more often. Think of it this way: Sometimes you're scared to death and do things anyway. Sometimes you find a way to be less scared. Those are two approaches to help yourself do the thing in front of you. All the High Vibe Habits contribute to this "dial tuning" method. Increasing your confidence levels allows you to approach life with more ease and energy because you are essentially taking down the hurdles, instead of having to jump them.

Overcoming Fear

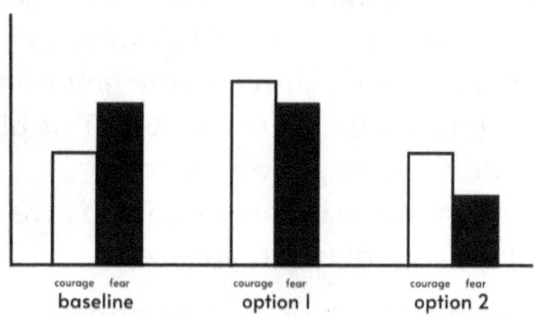

Chart 2 - Column one represents an example baseline. Column two shows your option I where you increase courage while fear stays the same as your baseline. Column 3 shows an alternative option where fear is reduced so brave action happens even without an increase in baseline courage.

We're more likely to throw ourselves into new situations when we aren't inhibited by fear. Unproductive thoughts diminish our confidence. Have you ever been super excited about something and then suddenly been stricken with fear as your mind started running through all the reasons why you should be afraid? Excitement and fear can feel similar in our bodies.

The High Vibe Habits are about decoding emotions for information, which adjusts the volume of our fearful thoughts. The scary thoughts are the ones we pay attention to, the ones that sound the most important (the squeaky wheel), and understandably so. We're designed to survive. But the modern landscape isn't fraught with predators and unknown terrain. We need to evolve to survive, and ideally thrive, in the emotionally challenging landscape we exist in. This place most often challenges our need for connection. We want our people to love us, accept us, admire us, and praise us.

The consistent focus on eliciting a fear response and following its recommended course of action slowly turns up the volume on this emotional dial. By default, the other voices inside us—yearning, hope, excitement, desire, possibility—all get drowned out. Like a sound technician, the confidence habit turns these emotional dials to bring them into a more melodic state. You're not turning anything off. The "dials" are habits that we learn to adjust by being aware of what we are over-, or under-, using. Fear still has a place, but amongst the other emotions, not over them.

When we are placed in an environment that feels new, our natural tendency towards fear and protection shifts us into another state completely. Even something as innocuous as sleeping in a hotel room can be enough to trigger your mental defense mechanics[14]. Think about how this affects how you show up for a meeting or a tough conversation. Needing to defend ourselves, our ideas and beliefs harnesses that same primal defensive brain power, making us less capable of tapping into the nuanced skills of empathy and negotiation. We're used to tuning into the discomfort and fear that occupy our headspace because we're wired to value survival skills. They are loud and send a lot of warning signal thoughts and symptoms to make sure we take notice.

This helps us understand why confidence feels situational and investigate how we can find ways to make ourselves feel more comfortable. We can stop being mad at ourselves for our lack and feel curious about how we can manipulate our thoughts to serve us. We want to cultivate a more supportive and productive thought pattern. Fear of the loss of love, safety, connection, and acceptance is so ingrained into our psyche

---

[14] Burgess, Matt. "Half Your Brain Stays Alert When You Sleep Somewhere New." *WIRED*, April 22, 2016. https://www.wired.com/story/brain-awake-while-sleeping/

that it takes intentional and repetitive acts to come out of our shells.

It's a very different feeling to be in a welcoming space versus being backed into a corner. The question is how do we simply return to being ourselves? It might just be a tuning issue. Sometimes all the logic in the world doesn't stop the voices in our heads shouting, *it won't work, I'm not good enough, everyone will laugh at me, people will think I'm selfish.* Fear is big, loud, and obnoxious so it gets our attention. Your other emotions will only get stronger when you give them time to be heard, seen, and validated. That's why it's so important to sit with your good feelings.

Overdoing

Overwhelm and exhaustion happen more when we aren't confident that our needs must also be met. Boundaries become difficult when we don't have an answer to the question: *what's enough?* We tend to take on more instead of evaluating what can be prioritized, delegated, or eliminated.

Boundaries don't have to be scary. Boundaries are clarity around what we want in our lives and what we believe we deserve. It's who we have to be to uphold those boundaries that feel uncomfortable. We think the uneasiness comes from outside, but it's an internal battle of beliefs: I am versus I'm not. Boundaries make us squeamish when our beliefs and desires challenge each other. Do you believe you are worthy of respect? We sometimes accept disrespectful behavior because we're not sure we're worth it, but we'd like to be.

The problem with living day in and day out with low energy is that you start making decisions from a low-energy state and that keeps you in your current life experience. The story doesn't change. Raising your energy and your state allows you to make decisions about where you want to be. And that lets you live the life you want.

Ever find it hard to turn off? Pause? Rest? Or take more than one deep breath at a time? Our "on" switch gets flipped and it's easy to forget that we have the power to toggle it in the other direction.

How do we answer that question *what's enough* without feeling guilty? We can turn this from a philosophical question into a practical one. *What's enough* has an answer when you stop and decide.

Writing this book gave me plenty of opportunities to practice answering this question. In the middle of writing this chapter, I found myself getting ready for bed and instinctively thought, *I didn't get enough writing in today.* I told my friend I wanted to get in another two hours. And then, I took stock. I had already completed one of those hours and had time for the other. I almost grudgingly gave in to the idea that I had done enough even though I had set a goal and was about to meet it.

Reflexes kick in so fast they're tricky to catch. Does your habit of diminishing how far you've come just because you reached your goal make you set a higher one? Or do you allow yourself to accept that you've done enough? What's something that you want to get done or needs to get done? What would feel like a good amount of time or progress for the day or week?

There can always be more to do. More revisions, ideas, and research. But when we thoughtfully set or even intuitively feel like we've met the requirement, hit the first target, or hit our limit, we can be done. One way an objective lens serves us is by making us better decision-makers. Growth and success don't require us to deprive ourselves of love and support. The end goal matters but so does how we get there.

Performance

There are a lot of factors that affect our confidence, all different faces of a single emotion—fear. Confidence comes when we stop factoring other people's responses into the way we show up. Our choices stop revolving around managing what other people will think, do, or say, and start coming from an authentic place within us. If you're using any distracted living elements like comparison or judgment on anyone else, chances are you're also using it on yourself.

Here's what fear does to your brain. You might experience confidence in one area of your life or maybe around certain people. As your comfort level grows, you feel safe. That allows you to relax and think and behave differently than you might otherwise. Think back to a time when you were caught off guard but couldn't think of the perfect response until hours later. Ever prepared for an interview or presentation and then felt like a deer in headlights? We've all experienced moments where our fear hijacked our minds.

I'm going to keep pointing this out, over and over because confidence is usually linked to performance or acceptance. If it's about pleasing, we tend to live reactively. We wait for someone to determine our next step. But if it's about being our best, we accomplish it through clarity, control, and confidence. We achieve and feel good.

Our thoughts determine our emotional state and that determines what parts of our brain we have access to. Our primitive brain developed around safety and basic operating functions. Optimal outcomes, productivity, and success are more likely when we are working from the forebrain of our minds. Our forebrain, the cerebrum, is the director of complex thoughts and function[15].

When our confidence is low, we wait for things to happen. Staying high vibe is

---

[15] National Institute of Neurological Disorders and Stroke. *"Brain Basics: Know Your Brain"*. n.d. https://www.ninds.nih.gov/health-information/public-education/brain-basics/brain-basics-know-your-brain.

empowering because you get to initiate change and growth. Essentially, you begin to ask for what you want and figure out how to get a yes.

There's a control-confidence cycle, one feeding into the other. When I exercise control, I harvest confidence. When I nurture my confidence, I'm better at taking control. Learned deprivation has us believing that confidence is an automatic result of doing, but it's not a guaranteed result.

Some degree of confidence is a byproduct of action, because the more we do something the less new it is. Practice provides ease and comfort. But with intentionality, there's so much more to gain. Yes, action offers us data to bolster our logical mind, but logic alone will never create the confidence level we ultimately seek. Confidence is a feeling, a self-perception, which means it's linked to what you believe. What you believe changes what you see.

Mondays are like New Year's for me—a fresh beginning. They hold for me the amped-up energy of possibility. Mondays, a day of dread for some as it signals another work week, are gifts to me.

How could I possibly love Mondays this much? My mother has always told me that good things happen on Mondays (the reasoning behind which is a whole other story). As a kid, I investigated. And sure enough, it turned out to be true. Now that I'm thinking about it, I did meet my husband on a Monday morning. On a subway car. In New York City. What are the chances? Mondays are good days.

Has this been true because I was on the lookout for something good, my antennae hyper-vigilant for an upward tick on my radar? Has it been true because random acts of loveliness fall on Mondays too? I wonder if it matters at all why it's true or if it only matters that I believe it to be true.

Our beliefs, often formed without a lot of thought or intention, are a force. Beliefs define us, shape our perspective, and attempt to predetermine our futures. This week, as you hear the chatter of your mind, listen. What do you believe? What do you say that maybe you don't believe? What would you like to believe?

Right now, just for a second, take a deep breath and let the word sink in.

Believe.

What do you feel? This single word makes me smile, gives me chills, fills me with confidence, and clears my worries. It's powerful stuff.

So, believe. In yourself, in magic, in dreams, in realities, in others, in love, in your why. Just believe. Get wrapped up in it. Let it take hold. Recognize it as a crucial component of your inner compass.

It matters what you believe.

How about you? What beliefs are you holding onto about yourself? About what you can or can't do? Good things happen on bad days and bad things on good days. In both instances, we create meaning from the state we're in. Think about the single incident of bumping your elbow. If it happens on a "bad" day, it can send your anger through the roof. "Ahhh! Why does this always happen!" And on a "good" day? You might just laugh it off. The life you experience is the one you focus on. Ignoring your strengths isn't humility. Knowing what you're strong at offers awareness of what you can keep improving. The steps you take in self-clarity will support you to see yourself through an objective lens.

Changing your perspective births new levels of confidence. You're not always the problem or lacking something. You have to be willing to see that you are a contributing factor to your success. Your control habit will serve as research for a data hunt. Reflect on what you've done. Your positive experiences are more profound and contribute to higher confidence when you ask your brain to take notice that you are in a feel-good state.

There's an ideal ratio of 5:1 positive to negative feedback that fosters a beneficial balance for confidence growth[16]. We can work to surround ourselves with peers, family, friends, and mentors who constructively support us, but we can also offer that to ourselves. Confidence isn't claiming to be what you're not. It's not overlooking all that you are. Being nice to yourself is important. How close do your thoughts get to that ratio?

---

[16] Folkman, Jack Zenger and Joseph. *"The Ideal Praise-to-Criticism Ratio."* Harvard Business Review, October 6, 2023 https://hbr.org/2013/03/the-ideal-praise-to-criticism

This is why, without reflection, action doesn't guarantee more confidence. I use the word cultivate with confidence because, for a lot of us, self-doubt and fear are our habits. Even when we accomplish things, we attribute it to something outside of us.

A big prerequisite for confidence is belief and trust, just as the definition states. Because confidence is a self-perception, you can look confident without being confident. You can also look confident without being capable. I think we all have seen incompetency delivered with confidence. You've probably also utilized some "fake it till you make it" attitude for perceived confidence. What we're trying to grow is our true confidence—belief and trust in ourselves, not just in our ability to perform a specific task. We're not judging approaches (that would be distracted living); we're learning to understand ourselves and our goals to make our success inevitable.

It's cool and dark, but I'm beginning to sweat a little. I tilt my head to catch a glimpse of the auditorium. The audience is a sea of blackness, but I know the seats are filled, my parents among them. The girl on stage stands poised in the blinding spotlight as she and the announcer go back and forth. Even though I'm next in line, the words they exchange are muffled by my thoughts.

When I heard about the Miss Junior Teen competition, I told my parents I wanted to enter to win scholarship money for college. But there was an additional push. At fifteen, I thought I should start to overcome my stage fright. No one else I knew seemed to find it as terrifying as I did, and I was determined to overcome my every fear.

"Aren't you nervous?" The girl behind me suddenly breaks my focus.

I look at her and calmly say, "No." She must've kept talking to me for a minute or so, but I can't remember what she said. I only remember holding onto that "No." Saying it aloud began to partially convince me that that truth must lie somewhere within me. It was "fake it till you make it" before I knew what that meant.

The next thing I knew, my name was called, and I glided onto the stage with the confidence of that "No" in my heart. Being on that stage was a showdown between who I hoped I could be and who I feared I was.

I won that pageant and the scholarship money. It would be one of many attempts, not all total successes, to battle the labels that claimed I wasn't good enough. Looking back, I wish I had been able to offer words of kindness that would have bolstered both myself *and* that girl behind me. Recognizing that that's the choice I would make today is growth I'm proud of.

Confidence isn't about changing someone else's mind; it's changing your own. That changed state of being alters the way you show up and influences everything around you.

Exploring Blocks

You might be noticing that the barriers to a high-vibe life are just a few fear-based blocks that are powerful enough to block many good habits from forming. Our past has set us up with a story designed by all our experiences and their outcomes. We know what we want to avoid and develop fears around the possibility of more pain. Remember that fear and faith are both choices that focus on what hasn't happened yet. That means a major obstacle isn't facing the consequence of our actions, it's facing the possibility of unwanted outcomes — *perceived* fear. It puts the universal needs we have as humans on the line: love, safety, and connection. Distinguishing between a real threat and focusing on a possible threat helps create a more objective lens to evaluate which habits support us. The following are new ways you can begin to cultivate your confidence.

Fear Is A Friend

Let's start shifting your state and redefining some terms. We all need courage when we face new things, but we don't want to keep drawing on our reserve. Depending on it is not a sustainable way to maintain forward momentum in our everyday lives. We want to work our way to confidence so that fear is put in its place as one of many sources of information we receive. Fear can become our friend. This choice lets us turn the fear dial down (see the chart above), which means we need less courage because it doesn't feel as scary.

I DON'T ALWAYS NEED MORE COURAGE. I CAN ALSO CHOOSE LESS FEAR.

When fear shows up, check in. Are you being served or being safe? The first thing to decide is if you're actually in danger. Then you're being served. Fear is doing its job. Fear serves us when we allow it to inform us of a constrictive belief. These lack type beliefs sounds like: *I'm not good enough. Not smart enough. Not qualified enough. There's not enough time or money.* This can show up as throat tightening, shoulders rising, tears flowing, or butterflies. All these physical symptoms are communication between our bodies and minds. If you're not actually in a dangerous situation, you have an opportunity in front of you. You can feel uncomfortable and step into the experience ahead and grow. You can decide to believe that new doesn't have to mean scary. Maybe you can let it mean exciting instead, an adventure ahead.

Reclaim Your State: Seek And Find

You change what you see by changing how you see. Most good days and bad days aren't created by what's happening around us. They happen because of what's going on inside us. Without intention, things that happen to us can trigger the story of a good day or a bad one. But living on purpose, being happy on purpose is about making that decision for yourself and leading yourself back to what you want. We can do this because our minds are programmed to run this way. Thanks to your reticular activating system (RAS), you find what you seek.

Now, let's apply this to confidence. What if you saw things differently? I'm guessing you spend a lot of your day calmly running on autopilot, getting work done, raising children, managing schedules, and planning. I encourage you to start taking note of how confidently you're moving through your day. Sit with that feeling on purpose. I'll bet you are accomplishing a lot already. There are a lot of moving parts involved in running a household and a family, growing a business, managing a career, or caring for your well-being. Anything and everything you're doing requires a skill set. And life experience is transferable.

I know the tendency is to brush off the daily tasks we do as something everyone does, but there's no limit to how many of us can possess a skill. Just because someone else can also do something doesn't mean it's not a skill. If you have trouble thinking of anything, what do people compliment you on? What do others notice? Practice thinking bigger. Above the act itself are general skills. Planning, time management, effective communication, and efficient execution are all skills you can use anywhere, including wherever you currently need a confidence boost. What if all the moments you aren't afraid are moments of confidence? I bet you'd find a lot of evidence to support the fact that you are more confident than you think.

Value

Here's a third perspective shift for you. Outcomes are for reflecting *on*, but not reflective *of* your value. If you want to be confident and build and maintain that confidence, you need to redefine your relationship with outcomes. We don't create value to be of value—it's a given. Learning to find value in your actions (there is always a gem to find), not flaws in your character will be the difference between forward momentum and going in circles. This mindset shift lets you strive for excellence. If in the end, you learn you need to acquire new skills, get more practice, or simply try again, do so objectively.

HIGH VIBE REFRAME

YOUR SUCCESS REFLECTS WHERE
YOU ARE ON YOUR JOURNEY,
NOT WHAT YOU'RE WORTH.

Here's another reason why needing proof of value is so futile. Proof of our value doesn't lead to fulfillment because there's never actually a point where we've done enough! Slow down and read that again. If you've ever hit your goal and didn't celebrate, listen up. You can't reach the finish line if it's always moving. Milestones can be short-lived wins because "enough" is relative. There will always be someone who is more, better, or farther than you are. Proving seems logic-based, but confidence is heavily heart-based through self-perception. If you don't see something in you, nothing you do will be able to offer you enough evidence. A drive to prove means that there's uncertainty, which, by definition, is the opposite of confidence (trust and belief).

Question whether your motivation is something that supports your growth or if it's something that validates your effort. Are you excited or exhausted by what you do? Life is a journey, and I believe in setting goals and achieving them. But the big-picture goal isn't about a finish line. It's about learning how to stay in the game.

The risk we run from not believing outcome and value are separate is a false sense of control, which can easily deflate our confidence. Adopting these High Vibe Habits releases you from the emotional roller coaster. You get to make constructive decisions regardless of your emotional state. You can capture the information that emotional state offers you (clarity), and then you take aligned action (control). If you focus on learning and growth, every step will breed confidence.

We get to let go of the old notions and images of confidence that come from outside of us and return to what we know to be true: Confidence is about having answers and asking questions. It's about speaking and listening. It's about leading and letting others lead. It comes from hitting our mark and learning from our mistakes. The certainty of confidence is in our ability to perform at our best (however imperfectly) and know it's a win because we can always be learning. High Vibe Habits are expansive. They make for an "and" life instead of an "either-or" one.

HIGH VIBE REFRAME

GROWTH IS THE TARGET YOU CAN
ALWAYS HIT.
PERFECT IS ONE YOU'LL ALMOST
ALWAYS MISS.

Decisions

I know it's easy to fall prey to this myth that you need to strive for perfection. We spend our whole lives living under the pressure of society, culture, and sometimes family to be good. These thoughts are apparent in our everyday choices.

Why do I feel like a Formula One racer when I go grocery shopping, eyeing the clock when I turn the car off and again when I hop back in? Because I get a great amount of pleasure when I'm efficient. Why? Because I'm more productive (and I used to believe that added to my worth). Productivity and efficiency still bring me joy, but because of what they make possible in my life. When life wasn't just about how much I got done, I began to see that I had other values as well. I was able to make space in my life for things like joy, living in the moment, and fun. The side effect of embracing all my values is a more balanced lifestyle, naturally avoiding burnout, fatigue, overwhelm and underwhelm (that's the 'there's got to be more to life' feeling you might get).

How about you? What do you do when you suddenly find yourself with thirty free minutes? Say you had an unexpected cancellation at the end of your day and the first thought that pops into your head is relief. You've been go-go-go all day and could really use a breather. The thought of going for a walk sounds tempting, but then you start to feel guilty. There are so many other things you could do with this time:

errands or that favor your daughter asked you for. In fact, there are a lot of "productive" ways you could be using your time.

None of these are bad. Confidence just lets us make choices from where we are instead of basing our choices on what others expect of us. How we view rest, how we define productivity (often linking our work to our worth), and whether we allow ourselves to receive what we need are all affected by our overall feeling of confidence. Taking care of your well-being is a good decision. When we are clouded by guilt to always be and do more, our decisions reflect that value system that doesn't value or make space for our needs.

Spend Time With Good Feelings

I'm guessing you're as good as I am at being able to nitpick about your life; at where you went wrong, could've done better, or fell short. The school of learned deprivation tells us the path to getting better is to focus on the bad stuff and breeze over the good stuff. There's no time for celebration before we move on. Just, *now what?* And, *what's next?*

Intentionally remaining with positive emotions and experiences for as long as possible shifts us into a more supportive thinking process and helps create a new habit. In *Resilient,* Dr. Rick Hanson explains that sitting with what's good initiates positive neuroplasticity in the brain. It creates a strong positive memory. We're familiar with our natural tendency to focus and ruminate on what goes wrong. The time you spend with negative emotions significantly outweighs the time you spend with positive emotions and thus becomes a habit.

Negativity bias is strengthened every time you use it. We're usually pretty aware of when we're feeling low, scared, or uncomfortable, but now I want you to create a new habit of noticing and spending time thinking about the moments, experiences, and decisions that make you feel good. That initial question, how do I feel right now, helps us out of a low place, but it also helps us notice our highs.

This C is about allowing yourself to feel all that good around you and within you. How often do you take the time to bask in your success? I mean this as a solo endeavor—a conversation you have with yourself that honestly assesses (that means judgment-free) your wins and your uniqueness.

Habitual behavior is practiced behavior. Changing your neural pathways to react supportively brings the ease that makes this a sustainable way of life. And the benefits don't stop there. It fosters inspiration and motivation. It also just makes you feel so freaking good. And when you're feeling good, you're spreading it and operating from a very different place—a heart-space versus just a headspace.

Confidence is greatly supported by action, which is why it comes after clarity and control. Why action? Because one way to create confidence is to prove perceived fear wrong. Positive experiences in turn create positive emotions in our mind. Positive neuroplasticity occurs from more and more of these experiences (the same is true of the reverse). How often have you done something uncomfortable and then thought, *huh, that wasn't as bad as I thought!* This is the proof we keep offering ourselves through repeated action—our perceived fear is worse than the reality. (In the next chapter we're going to talk about how to handle our thoughts when we don't like the outcomes.)

High-vibe states want to be shared. It's part of their expansive nature. Feeling good is an antidote to overthinking. Feeling good is contagious. Being energy conduits, when we have more energy, we give, do, and are more. And we do so with ease. You're operating from a space of wanting to make other people feel good. Your release from negative self-talk actually gives you access to a different part of your brain, an area that's far superior at idea generation, problem-solving, and efficiency. A great day for me at work makes me a better mother, wife, friend, and human. I'm even more cuddly with my dog when I feel good. I've heard it explained that gratitude and fear can't be felt at the same time. I'd add that most emotions that have us feeling good can't coexist with fear and low-vibe feelings.

CHOOSING TO STAY HIGH VIBE NATURALLY
KEEPS ME FROM LOW-VIBE EMOTIONS LIKE
FEAR, WORRY, GUILT, AND UNWORTHINESS.

The state of confidence we're looking to create within us is fostered by this feel-good place. We're more likely to approach something with a *why-not* attitude than a *what-if* one.

Take Imperfect Action

Even if it feels counterintuitive, taking action (even imperfect action) leads to more confidence if we reflect on it constructively. Confidence comes at the tail end of action and transitions you into the next stage of reflection. Our first instinct is to immediately talk about what went wrong or where we fell short. What we can do first, though, is identify what went right.

It's easy to gloss over (as it often does when we start out at something), but it's crucial to build and help our minds expand (strengthening our creativity) before we zero in on the typically longer list of negatives.

Last winter, my daughter had her first flute recital. She had practiced and felt so ready right up to the moment she needed to get dressed. Then all of a sudden, she didn't want to go. She wasn't thrilled about the idea of having a lot of eyes all on her. She told me she would perform at the next one.

It doesn't matter how old we are, our thoughts follow a similar pattern. We have the same thoughts that cycle on repeat. It takes new information to have new thoughts. But when we let our thoughts keep us stuck, we never get that new information. It's just a broken record of fear.

You might be excited to create a new vision for yourself, set new goals, or tackle something difficult. Keep this in mind as you dream up what's possible in your life and set your target. Don't let the old, looping ideas stop you from moving forward and getting new information. Fear might be loud right now, but other voices are waiting to be heard: excitement, joy, hope, desire, and they are equally deserving.

There isn't always enough practice to make us feel like we're prepared. Performance isn't about only preparedness, it's about the meaning of an outcome, how you define a result, and choosing an experience you want. For my daughter, the story of her fear was not the final story. She attended her recital and was proud of her performance.

HIGH VIBE REFRAME

CONFIDENCE INCREASES WITH ACTION AND GETS AMPLIFIED WHEN YOU RECOGNIZE YOU INITIATED IT.

You might be seeing a pattern within constructive living: It's an opportunity to redefine terms in a way that supports your growth. It's a way to feel sure-footed enough to keep expanding instead of stretching yourself thinner and thinner. A forward step always offers you a new perspective. Cutting yourself down is distracted living and offers you more of the same. You need new information for growth and to decrease your fear. Think upward and outward, like a tree from ground to sky.

Win-Learn

A benefit of constructive living is the new perspective of win-learn. This book in many ways is like a modern dictionary, transforming your language which in turn transforms your beliefs. Success. Failure. Achievement. Goal. Priorities. Joy. Rest. Fear. Courage. These words have all been defined for you, but their redefinition is part of the path to creating the life you want. That's not avoiding reality—it's creating your reality. Every situation can be seen from multiple angles. Instead of just asking if it is a success or failure, you can look for pieces of each. Win-learn feels better than the old win-lose. It sets you up to always be on an expansion track. You're either hitting your target or you're learning something valuable. You gain something either way.

I've referred to some universal sources of pressure: society, culture, and family. The pressure and messaging from those areas set our expectations of what's possible within us. Confidence is a boundary we uphold to relieve ourselves from that external pressure – a shield. It's how we hold space for ourselves. When you believe in yourself and possibility, you're saying an alternate path exists. I love this beautiful visual from Gabby Bernstein: "When an egg cracks from the outside, it's broken. When it cracks from the inside, it's reborn."

Live on purpose. When we choose to tackle things proactively, we do so from our strongest position. Waiting to hit the bottom means you're doing it from your most vulnerable place. Confidence grows with action, even imperfect action, because doing overcomes perceived fear and repetition helps us do it again and again with more ease. We harvest even more from that very same action when we practice the win-learn mindset and sit with the good, rewiring our brain's natural tendencies from negativity to positivity. Clarity and control lead us down the high-vibe path to confidence, where we make aligned decisions more easily and with less guilt. Feeling bad comes from feeling wrong. When our goals and actions line up, when we adopt healthy beliefs about our well-being, our choices benefit us and those around us.

Growth and success that don't require us to deprive ourselves of love and support build our confidence. Surround yourself with people who offer you this support and remember to always offer it to yourself. Being what we need and giving ourselves what we need creates a regenerative energy source within us to keep going and growing.

The first two C's strengthen your roots and tap into your true nature, desires, and potential. Confidence both roots you and helps you grow upwards. You've been building momentum from the beginning. Intentionally spending time reconnecting to your feelings, motivations, and reflexive tendencies (habits) all contribute to your confidence levels.

You belong in the life you want. What it takes to see it, create it, and live it often requires faith in ourselves and a loving, abundant Universe. I know how hard it is to show up, day after day. But don't be a stranger to the life you want. It can't feel like home until you spend time there. Beginning with your beliefs, thoughts, emotions, and then actions, feeling good can become natural and easy.

Here's the breakdown for confidence:

CONFIDENCE **eliminates**:
perfectionism, procrastination, stress, overwhelm, indecision, reactiveness, internal conflict, exhaustion, underwhelm, unhealthy competition, external pressure, regret, guilt

CONFIDENCE **encourages**:
healthy self-appraisal, guilt-free decision-making, aligned decisions,
growth, agency, perseverance, goal actualization, happiness, health, acceptance, responsiveness, self-appreciation, excellence, fulfillment, inspiration, empathy, patience, peace, prioritization

EXERCISES + INSIGHTS

Let's steep ourselves in confidence, practice this habit, and create space for ourselves to take courageous action.

Remember, confidence is as much about what you believe as what you know—your self-perception. It's connecting your action with new results and information. Cultivate it and harvest it through action and reflection.

Habit Stacking

Sometimes we need a nudge to push through the uncomfortable. Because you get to help yourself, you can implement habit stacking. It's a great way to remember to create a new habit and a way to treat yourself for doing something that feels like drudgery. Understanding your mental mechanics allows you to use them to your advantage. Seek pleasure, avoid pain—simple! Keep adding pleasure to your life. I think this has an exponential effect on your productivity and your joy. It's a positive snowball effect that will have you gaining momentum and building confidence in your abilities and your follow-through.

- Find something you're building a habit for. It could be exercise, healthy eating, or finishing a project.

You can do two things now:

- Find something that brings you joy and do it after your new habit. Each day you exercise, offer yourself a "treat." It could be reading time at night, a new workout class after a week of consistent workouts, or a coffee date with a friend. Find something that feels good.

- The other option helps you stay committed. If you find yourself procrastinating, tack on some amount of work to something existing in your schedule. I wrote a huge portion of this book by scheduling writing time after meditation. It could be tackling a clean-up project and investing thirty minutes toward it after breakfast on Saturdays. Tie something you need to get done to something you're already doing.

NOTES

Mama Bear

I've known from the moment I became a mother that I would do anything for my children. That included working on my personal growth to be my best and be intentional about what I passed on. Reframing any task in front of us to see our core motivation quickly shifts us into more confident action. Seeing ourselves as both students and teachers is a lens that reminds us that someone is always watching us. Maybe it's your children, maybe your sister, friend, or mother. Whether we are breaking ancestral habits or blazing completely new trails, we're almost always fighting to be an example for someone else.

Let these questions help you embrace your journey or allow you to release something.

- How does what you're doing light the way for someone else?
- How does it help someone learn how to see their full potential?
- How does it teach someone to overcome? To persevere?
- How does it teach someone to trust themselves?

NOTES

Follow this line of thinking when you feel like you're hitting the brakes, but what you really want is to forge onward.

What's Working

You know that feeling when you share something casually with your best friend and she's so excited about how amazing you are? That energy is contagious. It might get you thinking, *wait, maybe what I did is amazing.* Try creating that outside perspective for yourself.

- Make a list of all your wins! It doesn't matter how big or small—own it.
- Celebrate! It could be pride, or it could be a cupcake, just make sure you take stock of the distance you cover, not just the distance ahead of you.

You might find you're being the person you want to be and doing the things you want to do.

NOTES

Body Signals

Your body is part of an information feedback loop. Deciding how you stand and how deeply you breathe improves your confidence. Try this Superwoman pose:

- You'll take on the classic Superman pose, standing with your feet apart, hands on your hips, chest out, and head up.
- Stand this way for two minutes while breathing slow, deep breaths.
- If it feels natural, smile.

All of these signal safety to the brain. They're shown to increase your testosterone levels and bump your confidence up. Even if you can't do the full stance, keep your posture upright and stay in control of your breathing. Those deep breaths stimulate your vagus nerve and your parasympathetic nervous system, sending the "all safe" message to your brain. Remember a big part of low confidence comes from perceived fear. Get those confidence-inducing chemicals going instead of your stress response just by being in charge of your body.

NOTES

For more Confidence exercises, visit www.nithyakaria.com/highvibebook.

"

*What we think determines what
happens to us, so if we want to change
our lives, we need to stretch our minds.*

— *Wayne Dyer*

SIX

CURIOSITY + CREATIVITY

Did curiosity really kill the cat? I mean, did someone find the body? I'd like to think curiosity led that cat to a way better place where she's living an awesome life. My point is that if we don't dare to imagine more, we don't get more.

Remember that the High Vibe Habits help us first remove the obstacles we create to our happiness. There's very likely more of whatever you're looking for—health, happiness, success, love, connection—than you might currently be experiencing thanks to those blocks. The good news is you've been using these final two habits since the beginning. The fourth and fifth habits, curiosity and creativity, contribute greatly to the expansive nature of constructive living.

Clarity kicked us off to help us plan. Control led us to take aligned action. Confidence began rounding us out with a foothold in action and one in reflection. Curiosity and creativity are bringing us back full circle: curiosity is fully reflective, with creativity relying on our reflection capacity for idea generation (which helps us plan). I've been saying it all along; what we believe changes what we see. Not only do these two habits keep us expanding through their use, but they also exponentially increase our ability to stay high vibe because the blocks they remove are some of the most detrimental.

To understand how helpful they are, let's see what we use from learned deprivation. We find as many ways as possible to cut ourselves down; judgment, comparison, guilt, regret, and shame knock us down and keep us there. Low-vibe feelings can be interpreted as mild to extreme pain. Pain at low levels is distracting. Pain at high levels is destructive. I'm reviewing some of what we've already covered, but we're going to look at it from a slightly different angle.

Why did I start this chapter off with such a ridiculous question? We are told things, we hear things, and we infer things. But do we question them? When your mind gets into the habit of being inquisitive, you're always on the lookout for a new perspective. If you're too busy, too tired, or too distracted to do things differently, you'll always end up with more of the same.

Ever heard the story of the woman who always cooked her Thanksgiving turkey in two pans? One day her child asks her why.

"Tradition," she says. But the curious child wanted a better answer. So, she asks the child's grandmother.

"Tradition," she says. But now they're all getting a little curious. They go one more generation back to find out the child's great-great-grandmother did not have a pan big enough for their turkey, so she split it into two. . . and so the tradition began.

It's not about judging whether one pan or two pans is better. It's about keeping ourselves aware of what we do and why. Imagination is defined both as having new ideas and the ability to be resourceful. That means it can be applied in two directions. I call those two directions curiosity and creativity. When imagination questions, it's curiosity; when it answers, it's creativity. We need it for reflection: how can we see things differently? We need it for direction: what's possible in the future? Omitting imagination leaves us stuck. If you don't question what is, you're leaving a lot on the table.

Unpredictable, upsetting, and unwanted things happen. But when we have a habit of searching for multiple viewpoints, we can accept what has happened and find a healthy "what now." Buddhist teachings say that pain is like the first arrow that strikes. Suffering is the second, and avoidable, arrow that we allow to strike us. We aren't going to avoid all pain in life, but we can minimize the duration and intensity. The reason curiosity and creativity are able to rid us of suffering is that they offer us a new perspective. These last two C's allow us to ask ourselves what we can do, think, or say differently to create change. Dynamic thoughts create a more dynamic life. The High Vibe Habits do change things around us, but from change that happens within us.

Plan. Do. Review. We are just about done creating the full picture. I'm combining the last two habits into one chapter because they work synergistically—a dynamic duo.

Curiosity is how you approach a problem; creativity is how you find a solution. That will bump you back into clarity, where you will choose from all the possible futures to decide what best lines up with what you want. Prioritizing your well-being is hopefully, by now, starting to feel simpler and more possible. With time, it's also going to feel easier.

Now that you're not going around and around in circles focused on what's wrong or missing, you can feel free to investigate. If action is always leading you to new places, the High Vibe Habits lead you on an expedition where you always get to seek out how this all gets to work for you.

The *Oxford English Dictionary* definition for curiosity is, "The strong desire to know or learn something." It's a life approach. It's a positive inquiry. Curiosity doesn't put you down or make you feel bad. It's about learning, not about failing. The desire to learn trumps fear. Since our focus expands to include more than the need to categorize our efforts as simply loss or gain, curiosity turns our fear dial way down. Growth is the main driving force. We create meaning so this constructive lens changes the information coming in. And that changes everything afterward: your thoughts, emotions, and actions. Reflection can be the *I told you so* moment you have with yourself. Or it can be how you reimagine your future.

The *Oxford English Dictionary* defines creativity as, "The use of the imagination or original ideas, especially in the production of an artistic work." Can we pause here for a minute? This is not a skill just for artists. The life we want is our creative endeavor to bring together all the elements that help us live a full life. When you reread the definition from this perspective, you can begin to understand the role of creativity. Are you laying bricks or building a cathedral? Life will only ever be what you see.

Flip back to the distracted-constructive chart in Chapter Two. When we choose to follow the old habits, we lead ourselves down a more constricted path. Constructive choices lead us to expansion. Not just of our energy and emotions, but actual possibility. The state we're in ultimately leads to different decisions. Maybe you choose a donut over a salad, accept a so-so job instead of applying for that dream job, stay in your hometown instead of venturing out, or stay with the partner you have instead of searching for the one you deserve. No judgment on what's right or good, just awareness.

HIGH VIBE REFRAME

HOW YOU FEEL MATTERS.

Are you building the life you want or living distracted? Remember that distracted living keeps you busy believing you're making progress when you're really running in circles. The truth? Every day that you're living, you're either building the life you want or you're not. Studies show many of us end up having the same regrets in life. And that makes sense because even though our paths are unique, feeling good is a universal desire.

Looking at these common takebacks gives us a glimpse of what might bring any of us more fulfillment. People don't look back on their lives and wish they worked more or played it more safely. Risk and relationships rank pretty highly as areas people wished they invested in. All the High Vibe Habits support the mental state that makes you more willing and able to take the risks that will reap the rewards you're after. The best-self approach also lets us strengthen our connection to our children, partners, families, friends, and communities. A high-vibe lifestyle paves the way for us to thrive.

I believe one of the things that make achievement fulfilling is that you're engaging in the creative act of breathing life into something intangible (an idea, vision, desire) and making it tangible. I've experienced it and I've witnessed the excitement in others. Whether it's riding a bike or buying your dream home, it started within you and now it's something you can witness. That's powerful. And you've been doing it your whole life. How about that for building confidence?!

HIGH VIBE REFRAME

CURIOSITY AND CREATIVITY CHANGE HOW WE SEE, WHICH CHANGES WHAT WE SEE.

They are a huge part of the reflection process because this is the place where we most often cut ourselves down. Constructive awareness asks us how we can improve. Learned deprivation teaches us to focus on what went wrong. It's two sides of the same coin. Do you see what's lost or mine for gems? The stress distracted living creates within us diminishes the very skills that would help us be more successful: creativity, problem-solving, empathy, and memory recall. Practice win-win or win-learn instead of win-lose.

Best. Worst. I can often use these words to describe the same thing: entrepreneurship, marriage, parenting, homeschooling, cooking.

The things that matter most to me are often the things that are susceptible to the pendulum of my emotions because I invest so heavily in them. They are a big part of my journey and take up a huge chunk of my energy. I'm passionate about them and, in turn, passionately frustrated when things feel like they're not working.

I don't know about you, but sometimes when I'm running full steam ahead. . . I run straight into a wall. With all that enthusiasm for a new project, new year, or new idea, I lose my rhythm. When I throw too many things into the mix, I desperately need everything to go smoothly so I have the time, energy, and willpower to make it all happen.

But this is a quick way to forget that we don't, in fact, control anything beyond ourselves. The solution is one part strategy and one part perspective. Feeling down and feeling up is where we find our power or lose it. The dynamic duo habits guide our focus back to ourselves. It helps us manage our emotional state by choosing to let things out of our control go. Rather than let our feelings fester around blame, stress, hurt, or frustration, we can choose to revisit our role in things. We start with perspective because it shapes strategy.

Because constructive action builds new positive neural pathways, your new journey just needs your commitment. Small steps create big changes. Every feel-good decision you make is going to offer you proof and help you believe in the value of this work. The results will change your belief system. My clients have experienced this and so have I. Working on yourself will bring more out of the life you have. Every high-vibe choice you make replaces a distracted one and keeps you on your path. Maybe you want to be a great parent, maybe you want to grow a business. Personally, or professionally, we gain access to the skills that make it possible to hit our target more often.

HIGH VIBE REFRAME

DON'T STRESS ABOUT FUTURE DECISIONS.
GOOD DECISIONS IN THE PRESENT
TAKE YOU TO THE FUTURE YOU WANT.

One good decision leads to the next. So just focus on what's in front of you. The research by Mr. Sapolsky I mentioned a few chapters ago clearly shows that low-stress states are necessary for optimal outcomes. We lose access to critical thinking and executive functions under chronic stress conditions. It's not always that we can't get things done another way, it's that we are less equipped to do so and give our best. Distracted living feels hard and makes us work harder to be the person we want to be.

Curiosity and creativity have a childlike nature. They create space or separation between us and the outcome. It's a fascination with how things work, and it offers us an objective lens. Objectivity is the surest way to see possibility. Fear can blind us from seeing things that would bruise the ego and keep us safe from emotional pain.

Disappointment happens to all of us. I hear about it a lot around birthdays and holidays. I've experienced it, and so have my friends and clients. It might feel underwhelming, disappointing, or like experiencing the comparison blues. When I was a kid, my mother was extremely good at making me feel special, especially on birthdays. She was able to create a kind of magic around the day. I didn't know that was one of her superpowers until I got much older and didn't celebrate every birthday around her.

The idea of a climactic day like my birthday, Valentine's Day, Mother's Day, or even my anniversary, were days my mind would build up. The special day was often equated to disappointment. People's calls or texts asking how I celebrated were like salt being rubbed on a wound. I would cringe at having to tell people about my day because it was disappointing to say it out loud. I would see other people getting lavish gifts or doing something very orchestrated by their partners and feel deflated. The judgment and comparison clouded what I was gifted and how I was celebrated. I wanted to recreate the specialness inside me that my mother could always conjure up. And then I decided to get curious.

A few years ago, I noticed this old habit creeping up on me. I looked back and saw my pattern. I would imagine the lovely day I wanted. The emotions I would feel. The things people would do. And I would keep it all to myself because I expected my husband to know exactly what I wanted. This time I refused to feel disappointed. I wanted to break the cycle. I knew I had a good life, and I was not going to let myself take that away. As the calendar inched closer to Mother's Day, I took matters into my own hands. I got curious about my expectations.

Mothers are supremely powerful beings. (I say that more because I have a mother than the fact that I am a mother.) We get the chance to deeply impact people's lives. And not just any people, but those we love most dearly. How could all that love, effort, energy, determination, thoughtfulness, and so much more feel accounted for in a single day like Mother's Day?

Rather than be or feel disappointed, I chose to witness the appreciation each day. It was in the hugs, kisses, and notes. In the "I miss you" tears or the big "I feel safe around you" emotions. But most importantly I began to recognize my role in it all. I allowed myself to see my contribution to them and see the value in that work. I stopped needing other people's validation to know how amazing I am. Do I think it's important for other people to recognize that too? Yes. But like love languages, the people in my life (my husband and my children) were showing me their love and appreciation daily. Being celebrated is important. Learning you can celebrate yourself is important too.

Be sure you know how amazing you are. How valuable you are. How precious you are. How much you contribute. How worthy you are of all the great things the Universe has to offer. Create time in each day that's for you. You don't need to save it up for a single "official" day. You get to be seen by, appreciated by, and admired by yourself first. All the compliments, gratitude, and gestures from others are welcome but they are the icing on the cake. And you can always still ask for what you need.

I still love calendar holidays. But creativity offers me the gift of seeing the special in each day, creating it for myself, and communicating better so those around me aren't left to practice their mind-reading skills. Creativity showed me other futures were possible. I wasn't destined for a life of holiday disappointment. It reminded me of how to collaborate and create a life that feels good.

I GET TO ASK FOR WHAT I WANT AND I GET TO GIVE MYSELF WHAT I NEED.

You get to want what you want. If lavish gifts and dreamy vacations light you up, that's awesome. If a cozy night in by yourself is what calls to you, that's great too. Emotions are information. My emotions sending me into a low-vibe state were alerting me to a belief—that my emotional state was dependent on someone else's actions. I bypassed the idea that I could decide my value for myself. The comparison had me stuck thinking that love and appreciation looked a specific way. And let me also say this. The High Vibe Habits aren't a way for you to excuse other people's behavior or tolerate less in life. It's a path to exercising the control you have over yourself. Know what you need, offer it to yourself, *and* work through knowing what you want from others. Decide what your life gets to look like. As I have surrendered and dismantled disappointment blocks, I've been pleasantly surprised by 'special' days.

Rewiring supports our ability to feel good about ourselves and make good choices. The added benefit of healthy reflection habits is that they help us find more in the life we're living. Utilizing the High Vibe Habits, you get to feel good, make progress, and receive more from what you already have. That last piece is important because for many of us, what we have is at least partially what we want. Burnout, stress, exhaustion, and even underwhelm sometimes make us feel like we need to make huge changes. Curiosity lets us see things we previously overlooked. We see where we keep telling our old story and how we continue living that story on repeat. Creativity lets us feel excited to find all the other possibilities.

Curiosity and creativity buffer us from ourselves and other people. Limiting beliefs about ourselves creates limiting beliefs about others. What we do to ourselves (like judging), we do to others. Why? Because it's our habit. Constructive habits positively impact our relationships because our changed relationship with ourselves extends to everyone. When I practice curiosity towards my own emotions, I create distance and space so I can investigate and choose my meaning and truth. Making this my habit lets me reflexively apply this as a listener as well. So often the words of other people are rooted in the place they are in, not the place you are in.

"Sticks and stones may break my bones, but words will never hurt me."

Wow. That one takes me way back. All the way to the elementary school playground, a place where I attempted to use it as a shield. As juvenile as this saying is, I would search for comfort in its words for years.

In the end, it doesn't matter how old we get. It's good to feel a part of something, to be understood, and to be accepted. Whether it's the words of a schoolyard bully (with a flat-chested joke), a passing remark by a stranger ("your arms are hairy"), or an observation by a loved one ("you have big teeth"), we begin to transform into a guarded version of ourselves.

Daily interactions with others thicken our skin a bit, allowing some words to roll off our backs. But the ones that stick around change our inner landscape.

For many of us, the physical pain we suffer comes from accidents, adventures, or clumsiness. They are unpredictable events that originate from nowhere in particular. They don't feel personal.

Words, on the other hand, always stem from people. And they almost always feel personal. For a species that thrives on connection, acceptance, and love, words are a primary source of information.

With words, we define ourselves, find our people, take a stand, or inspire others. Words reinforce who we are. Words inspire. Words make us giants. With words, we feel pain, loneliness, or betrayal. Words cut us down. Words keep us small. Words plant seeds of doubt. Words deflate.

Words are powerful—choose them wisely.

When it comes to delivering a message, how we say things matters.

Words can be positive, negative, or neutral. Imagine how using the very same word creates different emotional experiences.

"Quiet!"

Spoken at a surprise birthday party gets everyone excited! The guest of honor is coming!

Spoken at a questioning child, makes her feel small, unimportant, and hurt.

Even an adult can suffer from this word. Imagine a husband watching a football game. His wife runs in to share an exciting piece of news. He shouts, "Quiet," and just like that she feels diminished and robbed of joy.

Words are powerful. But is all the power reserved for the speaker?

When it comes to receiving a message, we can feel powerless. Just as a spider's web catches much more than dinner, our minds become cluttered with a lot of word debris. I have spent years unpacking my pain and past, and the ickier parts are born from comments, passing phrases, and direct attacks.

So, here's my question.

Why do some things go in one ear and out the other, while others have a way of following us around? Why do some words so profoundly affect us that we give up our joy and opt not to dance, sing, or speak?

Here's my revelation, and those who know me have heard me say it before, what you believe matters.

It seems that words can become seeds planted in my brain. The ones that stick around begin to grow into something messy that tangles with my very being.

After a lot (and I mean a lot) of soul-searching, I have found my common denominator—two actually. My hurt is born from the truth, or from my fear of what might be the truth. The pain is my feelings of lack that get amplified.

Whew. That's a bitter pill to swallow. None of us want to believe that we think we might not be smart, beautiful, fun, cool, lovable, or funny. But I'll say it again: Almost all the remarks that have hurt me are ones I thought were true. Or ones I feared might be true. That's it.

When our truth is challenged, it's painful. Our truth is often a part of us that we can't, or *feel* like we can't, change. Whether it's our laugh, our bodies, or our dreams, we are exposed.

What do we do with this? The only thing we can—accept ourselves. Just. The. Way. We. Are.

This doesn't mean we cannot continue to grow and evolve as humans. It means that we are always being and becoming.

Most of us go out into the world as ourselves and slowly withdraw into our shells as we feel less and less safe to be who we are. We become a watered-down version of our colorful selves to avoid vulnerability.

But I'm here to challenge the idea that vulnerability has to be painful. Uncomfortable, yes, but with curiosity, maybe not painful. Our best defense is knowing who we really are so that when someone questions our character or motive, it is either true or not true.

If I find myself ruminating on a comment, it's an opportunity—a chance for me to know myself better. Now, when a word stings, I approach the discomfort differently. I ask myself: Why am I hurt? Is this true? Is this something I can change? Do I want it to be true? If it is me, can I do more than accept it—can I love this part of me?

I used to think my problem was that I wasn't enough "this" or needed to be more of "that." I used to think that if I could just take the best parts of people and become those things, I would feel secure, confident, and untouchable.

But it was exhausting, and I would inevitably fall short of my goal. My life was like a house of cards, ready to crash at any moment. Living in fear is draining. I also began to feel like I couldn't make any forward progress. It was like treading water when you could be swimming.

It wasn't until I got curious enough to look at my patterns that I was inspired to create change. High vibe let me have faith in who I was and where I found my full energy, optimism, and confidence return. Because in the end, we can never be great at being anything but ourselves. There is no trying anymore—only being, and the knowledge that I don't need to be all things. Just myself.

And you know what? The strangest things have begun to happen. Thanks to creativity, I found new strengths, new joys, and new opportunities. When I let go of mimicking others' successes, I found more of my own.

The kind that I'm not afraid I'll lose. The kind that doesn't make me feel like a fraud.

Sharing my voice has gone from scary and nerve-wracking to a way to create connection and joy. The transition feels like nothing short of miraculous. If you had told me all this several years ago, I would never have believed that I could achieve this kind of peace. But I have come to believe in believing, and I highly recommend it.

Exploring Blocks

Curiosity and creativity clear our vision. We come out of the fog that only lets us see a narrow scope of ourselves, our lives, and other people. In each chapter, we've gone over the thoughts and behaviors that block our way to what we want. Staying high vibe is first about what we can stop doing so we can truly see all that we can do.

Saving Joy

Later is not the only time for joy.

I'm curious, what do you love that you don't let yourself have or do? Do you own two pairs of pants in different colors, but always save the one you love for "later"? Do your favorite dishes stay safe in the cupboard for special occasions, or do you use them every day?

I have found Hello Kitty stickers from when I was in elementary school that I loved too much to use and now will never use. It's not about being impractical. It's about valuing today along with saving for tomorrow. I'm saying you can probably let yourself wear, do, or have that thing that brings you joy more often than you do. What are you afraid is going to happen if you let joy in every day? Happiness isn't fragile. You're not allotted a certain amount in one lifetime. It doesn't have to break the bank or mean you have to be irresponsible.

Creativity has helped me invest in a great stain remover so I can wear white more often. It's helped me find places where I'm spending money thoughtlessly and reinvest that into something meaningful. It's literally helped me be more creative because I let myself value downtime and see how joy decreased my stress and made me more productive. Creativity in the smallest ways leads us to a profoundly different way of living. Joy isn't something we have to save or something we earn. Practicing this fifth habit and following my joy has rewired my outlook in general. My new vantage point lets me include living enough in addition to doing enough.

HIGH VIBE REFRAME

JOY IS REASON ENOUGH.

Funny enough, as I type these words, I'm noticing that I'm wrapped in a blanket—but not my favorite blanket. I grabbed the ugly blanket! The one that I don't care if I drip tea on or if it spills onto the floor. Both blankets get the job done, but only one makes me smile. I'm going to get up now and make the swap. I love how curiosity keeps us observant.

Keeping Pace

Finding your pace doesn't mean you never get to change your pace. We often compare life to a race, but here's your reminder that it isn't actually one. So many of us set a pace for ourselves without understanding our motivation. I hope you've gotten curious about what's driven you to the point of not feeling good.

Maybe you're like me and hit the ground running, eager to prove yourself to the world. Having a career is often a heavy investment of our resources. And then we get married or choose a life partner. We have kids. And we're still running at the same frantic pace. It's what we know. It's also what we know is wearing us down. Curiosity opens the floodgates to: *Do I need to do it all? What matters to me? What's enough?* It's what lets us ask, *how can I make space for my health and happiness?* Finding a new pace isn't a sign of failure, it's a sign of awareness. The strategies of a marathon runner are not the same training, practice, or approach of a sprinter. Each goal requires its path for long-term success.

Curiosity applied gives clarity. What are *all* my values? You probably know the ones society deems worthy. But you can also check in and see what else you value: making memories, having fun, or being in nature. If it matters to you, it matters. Committing time, energy, and finances towards these values isn't wasteful, needless, or frivolous. It's actually productive. Learn to recognize all your values so you allow yourself to invest in them.

HIGH VIBE REFRAME

RECOGNIZING AND RESPECTING THAT MY ENERGY EBBS AND FLOWS IS A HIGH-VIBE, LONG-TERM SUCCESS STRATEGY.

We also get to permit ourselves to change our pace. Somewhere along the way, we pick the belief that we will and should always have the same amount of energy. But we each have a unique rhythm with an ebb and flow of energy. You run this course within a day, week, month, and year. You might recognize it when you call yourself a morning person or a night owl. You might notice you've got an extra bounce in your step during your favorite season. You might even notice how monthly hormonal fluctuations affect you. Respect your cycles. Working with them instead of against them helps you get more without feeling depleted. But you can't adhere to them if you aren't aware of them. Get curious.

Good Traits, Bad Habits

Responsible, hardworking, reliable, and generous. Ever noticed how these "good" traits lead to some "bad" feelings? You're not alone. Every single one of my clients (myself included) has experienced this.

We're praised early on for being so dependable, but then we wake up one day feeling like the weight of the world is on our shoulders. We're raised with short-term tools but inevitably find ourselves running a marathon. I'll bet you have a long list of compliment-worthy traits. Things you've learned along the way that get appreciated and praised. Getting in the habit of curiosity lets us see how often those very same "good" qualities lead to feeling poorly.

For most women I know, giving turns into over-giving. It's doing more, taking on an extra load (or two or three) because we can. Because we think it's part of the "deal" we made to have the life we have. It's a common distraction from focusing on our own needs.

The word "boundaries" makes a lot of us uncomfortable because it makes us responsible. It's not easy to buck the trend of playing the good-girl role that we've been raised to play. Curiosity pushes us into that discomfort zone (our growth zone) because we get to ask, *what does the person with these boundaries do?* Does she say, "Not right now," "No thank you," or just a plain "no"? Is she someone confident and willing to see, and accept, her value and not be influenced by others to do more?

HIGH VIBE REFRAME

BOUNDARIES AREN'T DIFFICULT, THEY JUST MAKE US UNCOMFORTABLE BECAUSE OF WHO WE HAVE TO BE TO UPHOLD THEM.

Working harder isn't the only answer available to you. As the "solution" to everyone's needs and problems, we lose the ability to meet our needs. This creates a cycle where we're all waiting for someone else to be the answer in our lives.

My eldest child has always been extremely capable and a quick learner. His

sweet disposition and eagerness to please
and make light of life make it easy for me to
forget that he's not older than he is. I'm sad
to say I've succumbed to societal
expectations of what he should be capable of.
I sometimes still find myself using the word
"should" while I'm trying to teach him how to
be self-aware. You "should" know when
you're hungry or tired so you can help
yourself, instead of taking it out on yourself
or someone else.

But then one day, I heard myself say this
and wondered (there's curiosity!) how often
do we, as adults, recognize what we need and
offer it to ourselves? Do you rest when you're
tired? Do you take care of yourself so you're
not tired? Do you eat when you're hungry or
work through lunch? Sometimes we're in
situations where we can't, but how often are
we in situations where we don't? How often
do we just keep driving, taking from our
reserves, until we get sick or tired, or so
exhausted we take it out on someone we
love? We live powering through life because
we were all taught at some level that needs
aren't information, they're luxuries.

Order, Schmorder

I'll be the first to admit it. I can fall prey to the my-way-or-the-highway attitude. I'm a systems girl. I love to think about how I can get more done in less time. I have an order and a process for everything. I love checking things off my list. It makes me feel good.

But it can have a few downfalls. This type of thinking is like convergent thinking — whittling down ideas and coming up with one solution. It goes against the divergent-thinking skills of curiosity and creativity, which let me see more options. There might be even better ways to do things. We're not always in the same place or moving at the same pace and believing there's one "best" way to be effective might not honor where we are in the present moment. The rigidity that makes this practice efficient is also the part that makes me stressed when things don't go according to plan. It's where judgment, comparison, and guilt can sneak in.

PRIORITIZING FEELING GOOD OFFERS YOU
MENTAL FLEXIBILITY TO SUPPORT YOURSELF
AND EVERYONE ELSE.

The other danger? It works amazingly for
my to-dos. But when it involves other people,
it gets sticky if they're not on board. Working
with others well requires us to see ourselves
as collaborators, not just taskmasters. The
point of being curious here isn't to discount
the value of efficiency. It's to check in and
value flexibility because questions are also
powerful and insightful.

One size may fit all, but it doesn't fit all
well. What works for your friend doesn't
necessarily work for you. When we look for
the right fit, we get to do a lot of trying on. It's
the exploratory nature of problem-solving.
We are capable of making a lot of things in
life work. But just because we can do it,
doesn't mean we need to do it. Still staying in
our judgment-free zone, we can use curiosity
to look at what's not working in our lives and
to get inspiration from other people. What

we tend to do is look around, compare ourselves, and decide that we need to do things like other people. Maybe it's about what a good marriage looks like; good parenting, hard work, or success. But not only are you allowed to find your way, but your way is likely to feel like it's serving you rather than you feeling like you're a slave to it. We each have our very own glass slipper waiting for us to slip into it.

HIGH VIBE REFRAME

I GET TO FIND
MY RIGHT FIT.

I understand why people have designated date nights, get their nails done, and host gatherings. I've also come to realize that the value of each of these things is different for each of us. Presentation of our life, our bodies, and our homes can become a burden if we do it all the same way. In my life, I've found that the list above can bring me joy, but can also bring me stress. Sometimes it's impractical, sometimes it's unpleasant. But when I've found my way to meet those underlying needs—connection, self-care, and community—they help me thrive.

Creating The Habit

I love looking at definitions as a way of reorienting myself. The *Oxford English Dictionary* defines curiosity as "a feeling of surprise mingled with admiration caused by something beautiful, unexpected, unfamiliar, or inexplicable." Doesn't that sound like a way better way to go through life than just seeing what's missing? Inevitably, using distracted elements to reflect on our lives makes us feel disappointed in ourselves, in others, or our experiences. Curiosity on the other hand lets us reflect with objectivity, which opens the door for kindness. Feeling hopeful about what we can change, or the fact that we can change at all leads to a feeling of wonder as we look forward. Being afraid of change or expecting disappointment is constricting. Wondering what's possible is expansive.

Creativity brings us full circle back to clarity. This consistently creates the most possibilities. Creativity is about generating as many ideas as possible and then running those ideas through the filter of clarity before you continue to cycle through the other C's and find yourself back at curiosity and creativity. These fourth and fifth habits build your divergent thinking skills. First, ask in how many ways can I see the situation. Next, ask how many possible next steps can I come up with. Divergent thinking is your ability to generate as many ideas or solutions as possible within a short period. It leads to expansive thinking and keeps pushing you to ask, *why not,* or *why can't this work for me?* This healthy forward thinking strengthens healthy reflection habits—a virtuous cycle.

An article in *The Harvard Business Review* talked about creativity as one of America's greatest resources from an economic standpoint. Without it, there's stagnation in our economy[17] and, I'm adding, in our lives. Life can feel routine, but even though there are a million ways we automate our days and interactions, it doesn't change the fact that there's value in questioning. As adults, our neural pathways are highly pruned from

---

[17] "America's Looming Creativity Crisis," Florida, Richard. *Harvard Business Review.* October 2004.
https://hbr.org/2004/10/americas-looming-creativity-crisis

running things day after day in the same way. My children are always reminding me how little I question whether the usual way is the best way. Or the fun way. Or if it's just *my* way.

Guess who else values creativity? George Land gave a fascinating TEDx Talk on the subject. NASA was looking for a better way to identify creative intelligence in individuals, a prized skill for an organization that wants to push the envelope of what's possible. The test was devised and administered to 1,600 school going children beginning at the age of five. A whopping ninety-eight percent scored as creative geniuses. The scientists tested the students again at ten, where thirty percent scored genius level; and again, at fifteen, where about twelve percent still scored at that high level. Adults came in at two percent. Why? Land attributes the sharp decline to our educational system. From a young age, we're encouraged to practice the thinking skills that encourage us to assess ideas *while* we're generating them[18].

---

[18] *"The Failure of Success,"* Land, George. TEDxTucson. December 2011. https://www.youtube.com/watch?v=ZfKMq-rYtnc&t=329s.

George Land and I use different language, but we're describing the same thing. He mentions blocks to creativity such as judgment, criticism, and censoring. He goes on to reveal findings similar to Robert Sapolsky's that we are losing access, in these fighting states (like the constrictive behaviors of learned deprivation), to the high-level thinking parts of our brain. We're taught to see creativity as a fluff skill, or one that's only good for artistic careers. But that's just another example of stuck thinking. If it's good enough for NASA, it's good enough for me.

Proactive Happiness

Why do we spend our energy trying to achieve something when it comes at the cost of something we value? We work so hard that we sacrifice our health. We are so busy doing it "all," we miss out on making the memories we long for later. How do we find a way to do what needs doing without sacrificing why we're doing it?

Happy on purpose is an agenda served by curiosity and creativity. That very first question we posed— *how do I feel*—tipped the curiosity domino that led to clarity. Creativity helps us answer the follow-up— *what can I do to feel better?* Proactive happiness looks like meeting your needs. All your needs, especially if they're not basic. Thrive and survive are two different paths. If you prioritize thriving, prioritize what it takes to get there. Meet those higher-level needs and microdose happiness. That begins with a pause and a question that lets you give yourself what you need. This process of initiating daily doses of feel-good actions leads to a high-vibe life and all the benefits that come with it.

Flexibility

Following the road less traveled is easier when we reduce stress around the unknown. Curiosity and creativity can be messy at times, but they can also breathe fresh air into our lives. Give yourself the grace to know when this approach makes sense. It's always beneficial to find ways to reduce your stress, but there's also your sanity to consider. There are exceptions, and stages in life—parenting young children, becoming caretakers, or investing in life changes—where it might be time to conserve your energy. But as a whole, it's generally beneficial to stay mentally limber.

Last Thanksgiving, my nine-year-old decided to create a secret breakfast recipe. She gave me a list of ingredients and then left me in the dark. Depending on the day, that kind of surrender can be hard for me. I felt my initial tendencies tugging at me. Was this going to mean extra clean-up time? What if her recipe didn't work—it seems like a waste of good food. I even started to feel ever-so-slightly irritated not knowing what she was doing, but still being expected to support her. Thankfully, I'd been practicing my High Vibe Habits, so those weren't the only thoughts I had.

Curiosity kicked in. I quickly saw the benefits far outweighed my concerns. What's the payoff? It's fortifying my daughter's confidence. It's teaching her to value the process (learning) over perfectionism (needing it to turn out right). We were going back and forth on finding the right kitchen tools when my son, who was listening, chimed in, "I'd probably just believe that it might not work and try something else." His words resonated with me.

"I would too," I said, thinking back to those first thoughts I had. I was so grateful to my daughter for sticking to trying things her way instead of mine. We all learned something valuable about ourselves. And in case you were wondering, her way worked! "Breakfast-dessert" turned out beautifully.

Feel Good Habits

Just because we can keep going, doesn't mean we should or that we have to. Irrespective of how you're wired, you can rewire. Needs aren't luxuries. When we treat them as such, we are bound for a low-vibe life. Sacrifice is sometimes called for, but it's not a lifestyle—it's a window. You already have what it takes to live the life you want. The High Vibe Habits help you make those aligned choices consistently, so your good habits are balanced and can support you and your loved ones.

Boundaries can be practiced in increments as well. Know what your decisions are costing you. This isn't about not helping others. Caring for your needs is how you help everyone else for as long as possible. Curiosity lets you gently pick apart what's happening now, and creativity lets you ask, *where's one small place where I could meet my needs?* That compassionate process can help you create more and more space until you reach the point where resentment and fatigue fall away, and you feel full and can give from that place.

Inspired Living

Finding your way to the things you want requires a big dose of creativity. Let there be joy in the process of exploration. Have fun exploring what lights you up, what connects you to your partner, what feels meaningful with your kids, and what feels doable when you give.

All healthy, deeply connected relationships take effort. Marriage is no different. Fifteen years of marriage feels like a drop in the bucket and a magnificent feat. It's very easy to fall into the it's-supposed-to-look-like-this boat. I depended on comparison to inform me on how to maintain a good marriage. And when it didn't feel possible, I assumed my relationship was paying the price for it.

Motherhood has been a very powerful and educational experience for me. And that includes how it's affected my relationship with my husband. I choose to invest heavily in my children, in the time I spend with them, and the attention I put towards their nurturing. I couldn't possibly know or understand the toll it would take on my body, my mind, and my marriage. While I courageously trusted my intuition, I also felt guilt. I felt "not enough." I felt exhausted by it all. I felt lost by how I could bridge my roles. For the longest time, it seemed like I had to choose between the things I wanted in life.

One of the most difficult pieces to fit in was how to continue to nurture my relationship with my husband. I kept watching other mothers happily carve out time for themselves and their marriages in ways that didn't resonate with me. I loved that they were meeting their needs, but I hadn't yet figured out a good way to meet all of mine. Curiosity and creativity have played such a big role in poking around for clarity and finding ways to take control.

In my mind, good marriages meant date nights. It's what we were supposed to be doing but weren't. There were a lot of reasons why. One of those reasons was that I'm not a night person. My husband comes alive in the evenings. I'm an early riser and prefer getting cozy at home in the evenings to going out late at night. I wanted to spend time with my husband, but I couldn't find the energy to do the same thing as everyone else. Did this mean we were doomed to a not-so-great marriage?

A few years ago, I came across a local park district volleyball class. It was an hour-and-a-half class, twice a week. That both my kids could attend. At the park a block away from our house. And it was forty dollars for fourteen weeks. It was a win-win-win. My husband and I walked the kids over that first Tuesday afternoon.

I was revved up to get home and get some work done when my husband looked over and asked, "What do you want to do"? I was totally surprised! He had worked out his schedule to take the hour-and-a-half off, and so began what became our routine day-date. We've explored the neighborhood for worthy outdoor patios, fun happy hour menus, and walking routes with beautiful homes. We found a way to spend time together that didn't pressure our budget, didn't require us to leave our kids with a sitter, and didn't need much planning. I'm grateful for my husband's imaginative thinking that let us find time together in a way that felt good for both of us.

Where do you maybe hold onto a picture in your mind of what some part of your life is supposed to look like? How can these last two habits help you see a picture of what you want it to look like?

Communication

Without curiosity and creativity, blame and frustration can become commonplace. Most of the time, we don't ask ourselves why we're emotional. Is it the dishes that upset you or is it that you asked for something, and your partner didn't step up? Could it be that you don't feel seen, heard, or valued? Being curious utilizes your confirmation bias powers. You have a filtering and filing system your brain uses to separate "important" information from all the millions of bits of "useless" information you receive. Use it to your advantage. The good news is when you begin to look for new things, you will find those too. Curiosity can train your mind to naturally identify your feelings and needs. That means you can communicate your emotions more effectively. It doesn't mean your partner or children will respond the way you want, but it does give you the practice to know what you want and figure out how to ask for it. It's truly eye-opening to see how many different ways we have the same conversation. Curiosity and creativity let us find a new angle with new information so we can begin to have more empathic and effective conversations. Try a new approach with these last two habits.

Those same conversations that don't lead to positive outcomes end up becoming either dangerously explosive or dangerously quiet. Most people I know who are in stuck relationships gravitate to one of these two extremes. Either each charged conversation ends in an explosion of emotions and words, or in a steely silence that cuts equally as deep. In either case, nothing changes. It's corroding a relationship that you most likely value. It's immensely difficult to show up differently in these situations because pride usually gets in the way.

Being right feels good; it validates our emotional experience and makes us feel seen. We want to avoid more pain. But here's the beauty of curiosity: You're not claiming guilt or innocence. You're not accusing either. The other person doesn't even need to be on board with this idea of change. When you show up differently, you've already changed the game. In a chess game, changing your move changes your opponent's options. It's like that in life as well. Anytime you do something new, something new is possible for the other person as well. You alone can change the dynamics of any situation. Taking control shows you the ball is always in your court when it comes to your choices.

We communicate because we want something: an answer, a voice, information, connection, or boundaries. And then we have an expectation. We act and we receive. What returns to us is technically unknown. But our actions have a boomerang effect. If people tend to act from the place they are in, know that your intentional actions have the power to help put them in a new place. Love, compassion, and understanding return different results than anger, hate, or apathy. I know how hard it is to change long-time dynamics. Just because one party is ready to make progress, doesn't mean the other one is. Curiosity gifts you the opportunity to change the place someone else is in without asking them to do any of the work. It's not always instant, but when you change what you see or what you do, you alter the landscape.

The way we present ourselves, our opinions, and our ideas are accepted or rejected based on how they're received. Delivery is vitally important to goal attainment because of the way it makes people feel. Curiosity and creativity remove the negative emotional charge behind interactions. Again, not because you don't have feelings, but because you want something different. Most of us learn to not express our feelings so we don't hurt someone else's. What we need to learn is that expressing ourselves doesn't have to hurt someone else. Understanding, and having empathy for someone, don't condone unwanted behavior. You still get to ask for what you want.

Reactive responses tend to be generated by our emotions. Anytime we feel under attack, scared, or nervous, our primary goal is usually safety and alleviation of that negative feeling. You might feel reactive and choose to fight or avoid. Either way, you're stuck in problem mode (the current one or a newly created one). In this mode, we become less adaptive and when the situation calls for creativity, it's simply not as available to us. When you choose curiosity and creativity, you're working towards the best possible outcome.

I had a client who had been married for over four decades. She and her husband had a set way of reacting and responding to each other. The heavily charged conversations they had left her feeling frustrated and misunderstood. Not long after working together, her new High Vibe Habits kicked in. Curiosity had her practicing empathy and noticing patterns. At a moment of high frustration, she remembered she could act from a more constructive place. So, she took a new approach.

She got clear on the points of her conversation and delivered them without accusing, raising her voice, or feeling defensive. She was amazed at the difference. In a very short time, instead of getting snapped at and called names, she had civil discussions and then pleasant ones. Her doomed marriage felt like it was evolving. A lot of big feelings, like loneliness and feeling unheard, began to be replaced by positive feelings that things could be different. Change wasn't happening overnight, but it was happening.

Fighting First Thoughts

When things go wrong, our minds are quick draws with negative thoughts. Confirmation of our fears comes crashing in proving our old story right. *I knew I'd mess this up. I'm not smart enough. I'm not qualified. I can't handle this kind of pressure.* With curiosity by your side, you can harness the power of objectivity to see what happened. Did you ask enough questions? Were you clear on the objective? Did you need to be more visible?

Instead of dissecting your personality and character, you get to do a play-by-play analysis of your decisions. You might witness the choices you made were shaped by your fears, insecurities, or misinformation, but curiosity offers you a learning lens. Being more visible means, you might get to work on courage and confidence. But reviewing outcomes and looking for specific, changeable action is different on our psyche than concluding we couldn't cut it. Do you see how you are flipping the script to tell yourself what you need to do, not what you lack?

What if you hate your job? Here's what curiosity sounds like: Instead of saying things like, *I'm stuck in a dead-end job* or *everyone else is doing meaningful work except me*, ask questions. What makes you hate it? Is it the work itself? The environment? The hours? Your boss? Now, reframe with creativity. Generate ideas where you initiate change. Instead of, *I want to stop hating my job*, try, *I'm going to apply to five new jobs in the next five months to see what my options are.* Or maybe, it's thinking through a conversation with your boss. Are you ready to up your game and invest in a new skill set to get you that promotion?

Asking questions transitions us from distracted living thoughts (constricting and fearful) into constructive living (expansive and possible). We've spent a lot of time talking about how a high vibe affects our communication skills and this is most powerful in the conversations we have with ourselves—the mental chatter. Don't worry, we all do it, talking ourselves into and out of things. Recognizing that you have an inner dialog is awareness.

Know Your Strengths

Your beliefs are writing the script for that private conversation. The simple act of objective thinking reframes what lies before you. You will start to see tools you can use and proof that you are capable. Then you'll start to hear your voices working for you instead of against you. Working from your strengths rather than feeling like you need to acquire someone else's is more effective and uplifting. None of us needs to be a patchwork quilt of other people's strengths. Know your strengths. Know what keeps you high vibe so you can access them. Creatively looking for a solution that utilizes your gifts is easier when you do these two things.

I've seen people use their sense of humor to diffuse unpleasant situations or make someone feel at ease. I've seen organizational skills kick in to override overwhelm. You can use your creativity to find equitable, peacemaking solutions. I've seen storytelling skills help people become better test-takers. You have strengths. And they can be creatively put to use in a lot of different ways.

If you're looking for guidance, I encourage you to explore the many different personality and strength assessments that are available. There's a list of some at the end of this chapter. One I found enlightening is a positive psychology assessment—Virtues in Action (VIA). Be open when taking any assessment. It's not a way to limit you. A test cannot by itself determine what you are or aren't. Use them to gain clarity. Apply curiosity to see how the results might serve you to understand yourself better. Get creative in their application.

One other trap to avoid is believing that there's a "better" skill or personality to have. I fell prey to this the first time I took the VIA survey. I browsed the site reading through their description of different traits and, without realizing it, was hoping I would have the "good" ones. I cringed a little bit when I saw that one of my top strengths was "Appreciation for Beauty and Excellence."

Not only had I never heard of this label when I first came across it, I'd also never considered it a skill.

I'm embarrassed to say that I took the somewhat lengthy assessment twice just to legitimize the results. That appreciation skill was there—both times. Once I accepted that this could help me know myself better, I dug in and was pleasantly surprised. I instantly recognized this tendency in me. I've always been drawn to both beauty and excellence. It explained my utter delight in beautiful things and my fascination with A-game performers. I've always wanted to contribute both these things to the world and reading about this virtue was connecting the dots for me.

It might be a person's compassion, charisma, or a physical skill set, like surgery or wood carving. I observed and absorbed ideas and inspiration by watching them. Before I saw this type of vision as a gift, I assumed I looked for it in others because I needed to learn what I didn't possess. Now, I know that I seek it as inspiration, a guiding light, to bring forth something already within me in a unique way. It's also shifted my state from envy or jealousy into true admiration and joy for the capability of the human spirit.

Get curious and creative with your strengths, skills, and perspective. Not sure what your strengths are? Pay attention to what people compliment you on. Take note of what comes easily to you.

Creative Living

I'm not creative. I hear this so often. Yes, there are a lot of people who are creative: actors, dancers, musicians, artists, designers. But creativity isn't limited to creative expression in these forms. It's a type of thinking.

HIGH VIBE REFRAME

CREATIVITY ISN'T ONLY ABOUT WHAT YOU PRODUCE, IT'S ABOUT HOW YOU THINK.

If curiosity constructively changes the information coming in, then creativity constructively changes what goes out: your responses, ideas, choices, and emotions. Your ability to alter what comes in affects your emotions, which affects your state. And your state affects everything in your life.

Strengthen your creative habit with your curious one. I know I'm not the only parent who's found an out-of-the-box solution for my child's problem (uncomfortable sock, broken toy, missing piece). Ever had to come up with something on the fly at work? Ever had a wardrobe malfunction and mended it on the go? There are so many examples of everyday creativity.

This goes way beyond parenthood. People find ways to live out their dreams all the time. We're just used to seeing the conventional path. Pick any life motivator as your place to start. How about a passion like travel? Some people ditch all their belongings and live out of a van. Some people work hard to splurge on luxury vacations. It's not wrong or right; it's simply choices.

We find ways to bring about what we desire, conventional or not. Whether it's a profession, passion, or lifestyle choice, there are many ways to have what we want. Instead of following the thoughts that tell us something isn't for us, find a new line of questioning. *how could this work for me?* Before you shoot down the ideas or inspiration you download, stay open.

Remember that analyzing ideas while we're generating them hinders our mental processes in all directions.

LIFE IS A CREATIVE ENDEAVOR OF TURNING YOUR THOUGHTS AND DREAMS INTO YOUR REALITY.

We bring the intangible to life. Now that's magic.

Let's be honest with ourselves. The tough stuff, the mean stuff, the hurtful stuff—sticks. That's the truth. But you don't have to believe it, hold on to it, or revolve your life around it. You choose your truth. Recognizing your old habits and built-in tendencies bolsters your healthy reflective habits. We can respect and appreciate our beautiful minds without condemning any parts of us as bad. Instead of classifying things as good or bad, we can ask if we are being served or if we are suffering. That's a more accurate, supportive, and useful metric to lead us to what we want—to feel good.

We're used to the good feelings not sticking around. It's time for a new normal. A high-vibe life is a filter. It takes the pressure off needing to be everything now and lets you feel good in this moment and see it as a stepping stone to what you want in the next.

The pen is in your hand. Author your story. A good day and a bad day aren't determined by what happens on the outside, but by what's happening on the inside. The dynamic duo habits in this chapter bypass our judgment circuitry. Instead of a defensive radar, we tune into self-knowledge and potential. Our brains don't need to protect us and trigger fear and stress if we see ourselves as in control. But how we see ourselves depends on how we reflect on our lives. With a high-vibe state, we shift from seeing our life one-dimensionally (the same old story) to a kaleidoscope of possibilities. Diminishing our resistance habits lets us exist in a colorful flow state more often. Achieving and feeling good.

Nothing wrong isn't the same thing as something right. What might you be waiting for before you decide you're ready to live high vibe? A lot of times in life we wait to initiate change until something is wrong, broken, lost, or gone. Working towards getting life to feel good, in that "right" direction, doesn't have to start with a huge undertaking. It just needs commitment to one decision—your desire to feel good.

It's tempting to leave good enough alone. If you're having some resistance to these habits, let go of the fear that looking back and getting curious about your life will mean you'll uncover something unpleasant. Up leveling doesn't have to be upheaval. Creativity doesn't leave anyone behind. High vibe is a judgment-free zone. We look back so we can move forward. If we only ever look forward, we run the risk of going in circles instead of moving onward and upward.

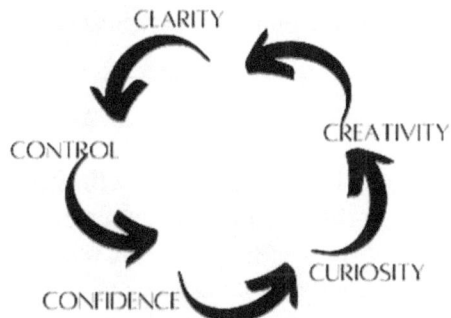

You will always be on an upward spiral as long as you continue to use each of the High Vibe Habits. All of us will have opportunity after opportunity to apply these C's because they are a lifestyle choice. Success, happiness, peace, joy—these are not endpoints, but beginnings. Borrow this statement: *I'm in training for the life I want.* When things get tough, I say this to myself. If this is your belief, how do you look at your past? What can you mine from it if it's all happening for you and not to you? Never stop questioning.

Here's the breakdown for curiosity and creativity:

CURIOSITY + CREATIVITY **encourages**: healthy self-appraisal, objectivity, possibility, hope, aligned decisions, growth, agency, goal actualization, happiness, health, acceptance, responsiveness, excellence, fulfillment, inspiration, empathy, patience, peace

---

CURIOSITY + CREATIVITY **eliminates**: judgment, criticism, making the same mistakes, perfectionism, stress, overwhelm, reactiveness, internal conflict, exhaustion, underwhelm, unhealthy competition, external pressure, regret, guilt

---

EXERCISES + INSIGHTS

Sometimes things don't go as planned and some emotions bubble up. Please let yourself feel them. Allow yourself to feel sad, bummed, or grieve if you need to. Just know that's the first step and not the last. Take a deep breath and when you're ready, curiosity and creativity will gently guide you back to what feels good.

Explore these two habits a little deeper. In your no-judgment zone, use them when something comes up or bonus points if you use them to relook at something that's working to see if it can get better!

Planning For Joy

When we get in the habit of waiting for something to make our day worth feeling "special," it can be very easy to end up waiting a very long time. Waiting for the precious moments automatically tells us that this moment is somehow less than another moment. Preciousness is a self-created concept. Bringing the nice plates out for guests reinforces that we're not enough to celebrate. Wearing the second-choice outfit encourages scarcity thinking. It might mean that getting dressed for ourselves isn't reason enough.

One of the best investments I made was in beautiful pajamas. I used to avoid spending money on things other people would never see. It seemed wasteful. But then I reframed. How can something that brings me joy be wasteful?

Remove your block to prioritizing and valuing what makes you happy. It doesn't have to be a monetary investment, but I'll encourage you to explore all areas you feel like you hold back in. We live in a creative economy where people are always creating more. Let's focus on the joy things will bring, instead of the fear that they will break, stain, or get used up.

- Get aware.
  Notice what you put off because it only makes sense to you or benefits you (like my nice pajamas). Give yourself the permission to invest and indulge in it. I started just browsing what I wanted. Then one year I bought a few pairs. The next year I bought a few more. Now, my pajama drawer and heart are full.

- Redefine special.
  What if you said Tuesdays were special and you decided to start wearing your favorite shoes or using your handmade bowls? Pick a day, time, or moment that happens regularly and make that the reason to do the things you normally wait to do.

It doesn't have to happen overnight. Begin to send yourself the signals that you and all the moments in life are precious.

NOTES

Best/Worst

If you find your mind goes to the worst-case scenario right away, this is a great exercise to gain perspective.

- Grab a piece of paper and make three columns

- Label them, "Best," "Worst," and "Most Likely"
- Under "Best," write down what your best possible outcome would be. Do the same for "Worst," but write what you most fear will happen.
- Under "Most Likely," get creative. What are all the possible scenarios that lay between best and worst?

Help yourself see that our first thought doesn't have to be our only thought. Most of the time what happens is neither best, nor worst—it's somewhere in between.

NOTES

What Could Be Better

This "Better" exercise uses curiosity instead of judgment to pinpoint where things could have been better instead of just seeing what went wrong. Awareness of where things went wrong is helpful when we know what we could do differently. We can learn even more by looking at it from the perspective of not only what flopped, but additionally what could be tweaked for further improvement. Placing ourselves in this habit of reflecting to learn removes that fear obstacle so it can become a habit.

- Pick a conversation or project, something to revisit
- Make three columns: "Goal," "This Time," and "Next Time." Objectively write what your goal was and what happened in the first two columns respectively.
- In the third column, practice curiosity and creativity to search for where you could use more high vibe. Investigate where you could have been more prepared, a better listener, or asked a question. This is not a judgment project. It's rewiring your brain to explore instead of cut down. It's also practice getting proactive about solutions and being prepared to make those happen.

NOTES

List Power

Just because you can, doesn't mean you should. Each of us gets to assess what works in our schedules, budgets, and lifestyles. Get curious about what's on your list. Delegation is useful but not always something we allow ourselves to do. But what if you looked at delegation, especially if it's paid labor, as an investment? What would that time open up for you? What would be possible? Could you make more money with your time? Improve your health? If it lowered your stress would that be good for your relationships?

You can do this exercise even when you prioritize. Even if you're not handing off the work to someone, maybe you can downgrade items on your list to make room for what might be more important or impactful.

Meditation and movement, for me, went from the bottom to the top of my list when I realized doing them actually helped me hit more of my goals. I'm a better everything when I'm of strong mind and body. Sometimes it means a little more disorder, but generally, it makes me more efficient and a whole lot happier. Check with your to-dos to see what can be prioritized differently, delegated, automated, and eliminated.

> NOTES

Password Playtime

This has been one of my all-time favorite creative feel-good tactics. It's the simplest little pick-me-up that bolsters my confidence and makes me smile. You're logging into stuff all the time so why not make it interesting?! (I don't recommend using this on anything you need high security around, like your bank account or credit cards.)

Change your password to something that helps you reinforce an idea that you'd like to embrace. Some ideas:

- Imarockstar!

- Bestmomever

- cre8ivegenius

- Cru$hingit!

The point is to get creative about what could make you feel good, smile, and support a positive belief shift. Keep changing them up as you go!

NOTES

For more Curiosity and Creativity exercises, visit www.nithyakaria.com/highvibebook.

"

It isn't about the pursuit of happiness.
It's about the happiness of pursuit.

— *Robert Sapolsky*

The ~~End~~ Beginning

Be impatient! Be so impatient when it comes to your happiness. There are so many things we must patiently tend to: raising children, having healthy marriages, growing businesses, planting gardens. But your happiness isn't one of them.

This unconventional advice, this whole book really, is meant to demystify, simplify, and systematize what we all want: to feel good.

The end goal of any desire is achieving it. And progress towards and achievement of a desire feels good. Joy is a universal aspiration. We're most successful at reaching any goal when we show up as the best version of ourselves. Living at the high-vibe end of the energy spectrum lets us be everything we want to be, and potentially need to be, in every role in life.

It might feel like you need everything to be perfect before you'll feel happy. But it's not true. Permission and pursuit are enough to make us feel good. Movement, momentum, and progress, however small, are enough. Joy isn't an endpoint, a thing you earn, or something someone gives you. It's a high-vibrational state of being. That means it's *how* we go through life, not where we're going. Everything we do and have can bring us joy. . . if we let it. Joy, happiness, fulfillment, and peace don't elude us—we filter them out by requiring them to meet impossible standards.

Living life relative to other people, or for other people, is like aiming at a moving target. How you feel doesn't need to be dependent on someone or something else. Learned deprivation through comparison, guilt, judgment, regret, or shame leaves us feeling stuck, lacking, lonely, and unworthy because we're working in a low-vibe cycle. These conditioned habits block our ability to see the good that exists, as well as deny us the potential for more. Sacrifice is doable and sometimes necessary. But it's an act, not a lifestyle. If you are always giving up a piece of yourself, you downgrade your life with negative thoughts and emotions. The things that bring you joy start to deplete you. What you want isn't the problem. It's just not fair to expect a life that was never built to account for your needs to be able to suddenly do so. Your new goal needs a new way. Thriving requires a different approach than surviving.

The goal isn't to stop doing for others but to start consistently doing for yourself. That's how you give more, over and over again. Quality, not just quantity, because you become an energy conduit. What you invest in yourself, you pass on to others. You don't give yourself; you give *of* yourself. Learning to receive lets each of us become proactive about our emotional state knowing what we need and offering it to ourselves. It matters what you believe because it changes how you feel. How you feel (your energetic vibrational state) affects every thought you have and every decision you make.

The information we feel like we need to know to feel safe, happy, secure, and connected is actually less necessary than we think. What we need changes when we gift ourselves love, acceptance, and worthiness. The answer to whether *will I find the love of my life* matters less than *whether I can love myself.* The answer to whether *will I be successful* matters less than believing *success is something I define for myself.* The answer to *will I have a great relationship with my children* is better answered by *will I make the choices that make great relationships possible.* The answers we hope for are the futures we hope for. The tomorrow we want is decided in the moment we're in. If we are making aligned decisions in the small moments, we are all always moving closer to the future we want.

Ask the right questions:

- How am I feeling right now?
- What are those feelings telling me?
- What could I do to feel better? (microdosing happiness)
- What parts of my life feel good? What parts don't?
- What small thing could I do today to move me towards my goal?
- What are my strengths?
- What did I learn?
- Where can I grow?
- What could I have done differently?
- What could I do or try next time?

These questions reflect the High Vibe Habits. The High Vibe Habits are in the questions. They're habits that help us create momentum by encouraging us to be intentional, to take imperfect action, and to see how it works out for us. Know where you stand at any given moment. If you're in a low place, start with these questions. Climb your way to a higher-vibe state with these five habits. Your value is a given, but growth is a choice.

As children, we live in a state of joy. It gets trained out of us as we grow up. As women, if we aren't considering someone else, our guilt reflex easily kicks in. We neglect our bodies and our minds because prioritizing ourselves means doing something that's just for us. We know taking care of ourselves helps us take care of others. But each of us has created a life that squeezed out our needs to make space for being all the things we're expected to be. For a lot of us, that's perfect.

We try to do all the things. When our needs get bumped down the list or off our calendars, we cut ourselves down believing we lack what it takes. We're not avoiding sleep, eating poorly, being sedentary, or denying ourselves joy because we're poor at managing our time or don't have enough resources. We do these things because we've been habituated to the idea that we're only allowed to give and do. None of us will reallocate our resources (time, money, energy) until we believe in our value and realize we are an important contributing being to the life we've built.

The fact that we've been, or are, successful perpetuates the idea that we're somehow the problem. Like if we've done it before, we should be able to keep doing it. So, we work harder. But you don't have to lose yourself to win at life. Small, consistent steps towards feeling good begin a cycle of infinite possibility.

I used to think that people who were happy, healthy, and vibrant were that way because their life was easier than mine. The truth is that happiness, health, and joy are values people commit to. They have clarity, take control, and confidently move towards a life they want.

Did you know that Earth lies in what scientists call a "Goldilocks Zone"? It's like the fable; we're just the right distance (not too close or too far) from the sun to sustain an abundance of life. I believe we all get to find our "Goldilocks Zone"—that just right place where we flourish. We all want to head to the feel-good zone. That magical life looks different for each of us. But what is the same for us all is what it doesn't include: deprivation, lack, fear, neglect, or low vibe living. It's a state of more: more energy, more time, more confidence, more joy, more to give. When you have more, you give more. Whatever you're hoping to accomplish in this lifetime will be supported by this place.

The High Vibe Habits keep you happy on purpose. Feeling good still isn't widely considered a valuable goal. But you've just read some of the science behind the power of a high-vibe state of being. And you've got your intuition to back it up. You know you can't be in two places at once; neither can your emotions. You can't be upset and curious, jealous and inspired, or miserable and grateful at the same time. Proactive happiness is your choosing which end of the energetic continuum you're on. One of love and possibility or one of fear and lack. Focusing your efforts on a high-vibe lifestyle offers you the pleasant side effects of less stress, more joy, better health, more success, and more ease.

Fear's presence doesn't mean you're not supposed to do the thing, take the leap, or make a stand. Fear says you're on the edge. Its presence signifies the potential for expansion. So, expand, get bigger, take up more room. Keep fear by your side like a trusted advisor pointing you in the direction of your next greatest move. Don't condemn who you are, learn to harness the power of all your emotions.

You are valuable simply because you exist.

My nine-year-old daughter and ninety-nine-year-old grandmother, two of the strongest females I know, have shared similar sentiments with me: feeling like they aren't valued. When we're young, we go around proving ourselves worthy to gain respect, experience, and confidence. Learning a skill is how we contribute to the world, not how we prove our value. Your work is not your worth.

As we age, we often feel our declining contributions and abilities mean a decline in our value and worth. Let's bust this myth too, please. I don't want anyone to believe that they are nothing but a burden. Our presence, our life force, has the ability to bring joy, peace, companionship, laughter, and love. Those are some of the most magnificent gifts we can offer at any point in our lives. Passing through different stages sometimes makes us dependent on others but never changes our value. Your work is not your worth.

I'm somewhere in the middle and have found myself wrestling with this same demon. You aren't here to prove yourself. You're here to bring forth what lies within you and create the life you envision. Checking off your to-do list, earning a salary, and performing household duties reflect types of contribution. Your worth isn't dependent on your income, family size, address, or accolades. Never feel diminished.

Do this for you. But if that feels too difficult, do it for someone else. I know how easy it is to overlook the influence you have on the world around you. But someone is always watching. Even if you're not on a big stage, you're impacting lives. I know it's easier to find courage when you do things for someone else. I hope you realize you are worth this work, but I also know how deeply beliefs can run. The habit of loving yourself enough to be the reason is truly the best way to give everyone around you the permission to do the same—value themselves.

Start microdosing happiness today. Do the small acts of kindness, remove the feel-good obstacles, and ask the loving question: *how do I feel right now?* And always remember, the answer matters. You matter. You get to want what you want. Period. Feeling good is reason enough. Wherever you are, you're only a few habits away from making joy your reflex.

All the High Vibe Habits are already a part of you. You are learning to lean on them to draw out the power within you. As your go-to habits, you can follow your feel-good North Star and lead the life you envision. By implementing this microdosing happiness "drip" system, you avoid the places that become difficult to escape from like guilt, regret, burnout, underwhelm, exhaustion, and chronic stress, simply by allowing yourself to focus on feeling good daily. That elevated state guides you to make one good decision after another. The life you experience is just a series of single steps that either lead you to hope or away from it. Hope leads you to possibility. The High Vibe Habits expand you further, turning possibility into probability.

Don't find time. Create it. Prioritizing your health and happiness benefits everyone. We shouldn't need science to prove what we intuitively know. We matter. Taking care of ourselves makes a difference. Others' benefiting from our work is a part of the virtuous well-being cycle. Feeling good raises your vibrational state and expands you. And it takes so much less to get there than you think. Consistency is key. And it's easier with the right habits.

The simplicity of the solution doesn't change the reality that our beliefs are deeply rooted within us. Retraining our minds and replacing old thoughts requires us to first show up with love and compassion for ourselves. We can't muscle our way to high vibe. We surrender, shed, and love our way there.

Remember, you can pour into your life, but if you don't let it pour back into you it's difficult to feel fulfilled. Achievement is based on your ability to give. Happiness is based on your ability to receive. With the

High Vibe Habits, you can give and receive, achieve and feel good.

The High Vibe Habits' complementary and compounding nature means you can (and will want to) use them simultaneously. You began by creating a map and finding your place (clarity). You've taken steps to move you towards your goal (control). You began reflecting on your wins and strengths (confidence). In the last chapter, we walked through how to objectively reflect on your actions, review your missteps with curiosity, and choose to harvest the lessons for forward progress. Asking better questions makes you better at making future choices that produce desired outcomes. Creativity opens your mind up to new ideas and possibilities for what lies ahead. It feeds back into your clarity, completing the circle. Even though you will return to the same C's, you will never be in the same place.

The High Vibe Habits offer you all three: the destination, the directions, and the discipline. I want this book to carry more than hope. This book is meant to guide you back to what you need to succeed in the life of your choice. Those happy, healthy people you see simply prioritize what it takes to stay that way. They're in the habit of feeling good.

You already have everything you need to create the life you want. You simply need a way to draw it out of you. I hear some version of this all the time: *I don't have time to feel good.* You don't have time *not* to feel good! You might think it's expensive to invest in what you need. But your life is already costing you more precious things: memories, peace, relationships, your health and longevity—your happiness! All of these, any of these, are worthy goals. The last one especially. Feeling good isn't an expensive state, it's an expansive one.

This isn't "the end." My hope is for you to see this as a beginning. Every moment is. This holds true when things go well and when times are tough. There's more to come. The next moment is here. Choose it. Choose you.

I'm rooting for you. Stay high vibe, my friend.

With all my love and gratitude,

Nithya

ACKNOWLEDGEMENTS

I have been blessed by a great many people. Thank you to each and every one of you who have reinforced that the world is a good place and that it's filled with good people. You help me believe in high vibe.

Thank you to all the researchers, scientists, spiritual leaders, doctors, coaches and authors who share their work and teach me so much. You inspire me to stay curious and flexible.

Thank you to my coach Sara, the editors and the whole team at Muse for getting this out of me and into the world.

I feel especially called to thank five women who have powerfully and lovingly shaped me. For me to say this book is a piece of me is to say that you five have played a role in its making. I love you all fiercely.

Amma, you have always been my dreamcatcher. Your impact on my life is unmatched. Thank you for showing me that I can also be my own dreamcatcher. Mallichithi, your love and unending support

are like an eternal flame that warms my soul
and lights my way. Ammamma, we have
always been two souls as one, bound by love.
You are the greatest example of love,
strength, and faith I have ever known. I am
unbelievably blessed to have you as my
grandmother. Thank you for absolutely
everything.

To my besties, D and H, forty years
together has created so much more than
friendship. The laughter, looks, love, and
tears we have shared bound us deeply and
forged a sisterhood for which I am eternally
grateful.

Gautam - You are my rock and have
helped make the life I live possible. Thank
you for always loving me, supporting me, and
helping me grow, but most of all thank you
for always knowing how to make me laugh.
You are my love story.

And of course, to my little ones. I am
beyond blessed to be your Amma. I could not
have fathomed how being your mother
would shape me. You are my everything.
Thank you for your patience, love, support,
and editing skills as I envisioned, wrote, and
rewrote this book. Thank you for your loving
words of encouragement and for believing in

me without a doubt. I love you to the moon
and back.

AUTHOR BIO

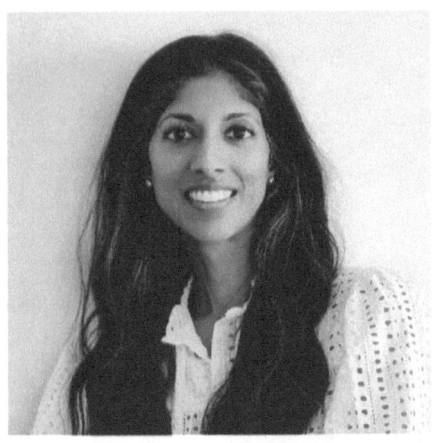

Nithya Karia is an author, coach, and creative entrepreneur with nearly fifteen years of experience guiding individuals and organizations toward simpler, more stress-free living. In a world where juggling motherhood, marriage, work, and personal satisfaction can feel overwhelming, Nithya offers a refreshing approach to wellness. Blending science with intuitive wisdom, she reveals the transformative power of simply feeling good. Her practical approach isn't hinged on denying others' needs, but in building a life that can meet yours as well. Her philosophy? When we take care of ourselves first, everything else falls into place—creating what she calls a "champagne-tower life."